T0263276

Geriatric Medicine

Editor

CATHERINE M. MCGOWAN

VETERINARY CLINICS OF NORTH AMERICA: EQUINE PRACTICE

www.vetequine.theclinics.com

Consulting Editor
THOMAS J. DIVERS

August 2016 • Volume 32 • Number 2

ELSEVIER

1600 John F. Kennedy Boulevard • Suite 1800 • Philadelphia, Pennsylvania, 19103-2899

http://www.vetequine.theclinics.com

VETERINARY CLINICS OF NORTH AMERICA: EQUINE PRACTICE Volume 32, Number 2
August 2016 ISSN 0749-0739, ISBN-13: 978-0-323-45995-2

Editor: Patrick Manley
Developmental Editor: Donald Mumford

Veterinary Clinics of North America: Equine Practice (ISSN 0749-0739) is published in April, August, and December by Elsevier Inc., 360 Park Avenue South, New York, NY 10010-1710. Business and Editorial Offices: 1600 John F. Kennedy Blvd., Suite 1800, Philadelphia, PA 19103-2899. Subscription prices are $270.00 per year (domestic individuals), $477.00 per year (domestic institutions), $100.00 per year (domestic students/residents), $315.00 per year (Canadian individuals), $601.00 per year (Canadian institutions), $365.00 per year (international individuals), $601.00 per year (international institutions), and $180.00 per year (international and Canadian students/residents). To receive student/resident rate, orders must be accompanied by name of affiliated institution, date of term, and the signature of program/residency coordinator on institution letterhead. Orders will be billed at individual rate until proof of status is received. Foreign air speed delivery is included in all *Clinics* subscription prices. All prices are subject to change without notice. **POSTMASTER:** Send address changes to *Veterinary Clinics of North America: Equine Practice*, 3251 Riverport Lane, Maryland Heights, MO 63043. Customer Service (orders, claims, online, change of address): Elsevier Health Sciences Division, Subscription **Customer Service, 3251 Riverport Lane, Maryland Heights, MO 63043. Tel: 1-800-654-2452 (U.S. and Canada); 314-447-8871 (outside U.S. and Canada). Fax: 314-447-8029. E-mail: journalscustomerservice-usa@elsevier.com (for print support);** E-mail: **journalsonlinesupport-usa@elsevier. com (for online support)**.

Reprints. For copies of 100 or more of articles in this publication, please contact the Commercial Reprints Department, Elsevier Inc., 360 Park Avenue South, New York, NY 10010-1710. Tel.: 212-633-3874; Fax: 212-633-3820; E-mail: reprints@elsevier.com.

Veterinary Clinics of North America: Equine Practice is covered in *MEDLINE/PubMed (Index Medicus)*, *Excerpta Medica, Current Contents/Agriculture, Biology and Environmental Sciences*, and *ISI*.

Contributors

CONSULTING EDITOR

THOMAS J. DIVERS, DVM
Diplomate, American College of Veterinary Internal Medicine; Diplomate, American
College of Veterinary Emergency and Critical Care; Steffen Professor of Veterinary
Medicine, Section Chief, Section of Large Animal Medicine, College of Veterinary
Medicine, Cornell University, Ithaca, New York

EDITOR

CATHERINE M. McGOWAN, BVSc, MACVS, PhD, FHEA, MRCVS
Diploma in Equine Internal Medicine; Diplomate, European College of Equine Internal
Medicine; Head of Equine and Director of Veterinary Postgraduate Education, Professor of
Equine Internal Medicine, Faculty of Health and Life Sciences, Institute of Ageing and
Chronic Disease and Institute of Veterinary Science, University of Liverpool, Wirral,
United Kingdom

AUTHORS

CAROLINE McG. ARGO, BSc, BVSc, PhD, MRCVS
Diplomate of the European College of Animal Reproduction; Department of Veterinary
Clinical Sciences, School of Veterinary Medicine, Faculty of Health and Medical Sciences,
University of Surrey, Guildford, United Kingdom

WILLEM BACK, DVM, PhD
Diplomate, European College of Veterinary Surgeons; Department of Equine Sciences,
Faculty of Veterinary Medicine, Utrecht University, Utrecht, the Netherlands; Department
of Surgery and Anaesthesiology, Faculty of Veterinary Medicine, Ghent University,
Merelbeke, Belgium

ANDY E. DURHAM, BSc, BVSc, CertEP, MRCVS
Royal College of Veterinary Surgeons' Diploma in Equine Internal Medicine; Diplomate,
European College of Equine Internal Medicine; Professor, Liphook Equine Hospital,
Liphook, Hampshire, United Kingdom

JOANNE L. IRELAND, BVMS, PhD, Cert AVP(EM), MRCVS
Epidemiologist, Epidemiology and Disease Surveillance, Centre for Preventive Medicine,
Animal Health Trust, Newmarket, Suffolk, United Kingdom

DEREK C. KNOTTENBELT, OBE, BVM&S, DVM&S, MRCVS
Diplomate, European College of Equine Internal Medicine; Consultant in Equine Internal
Medicine, RCVS and European Recognized Specialist, Equine Internal Medicine,
University of Glasgow, Glasgow, Scotland

FERNANDO MALALANA, DVM, FHEA, MRCVS
Diplomate, European College of Equine Internal Medicine; Philip Leverhulme Equine
Hospital, University of Liverpool, Neston, United Kingdom

CELIA M. MARR, BVMS, MVM, PhD
Diplomate, European College of Equine Internal Medicine; Rossdales Equine Hospital and Diagnostic Centre, Suffolk, United Kingdom

DIANNE McFARLANE, DVM, PhD
Diplomate, American College of Veterinary Internal Medicine; Department of Physiological Sciences, Center of Veterinary Health Sciences, Stillwater, Oklahoma

CATHERINE M. McGOWAN, BVSc, MACVS, PhD, FHEA, MRCVS
Diploma in Equine Internal Medicine; Diplomate, European College of Equine Internal Medicine; Head of Equine and Director of Veterinary Postgraduate Education, Professor of Equine Internal Medicine, Faculty of Health and Life Sciences, Institute of Ageing and Chronic Disease and Institute of Veterinary Science, University of Liverpool, Wirral, United Kingdom

KENNETH HARRINGTON McKEEVER, MS, PhD, FACSM
Department of Animal Science, Professor of Equine Exercise Physiology, Equine Science Center, School of Environmental and Biological Sciences, Rutgers, the State University of New Jersey, New Brunswick, New Jersey

VICTORIA M. NICHOLLS, BSc (Hons), BVetMed, Cert AVP (EM), Cert AVP (ED), MRCVS
Veterinary Postgraduate Unit, University of Liverpool, School of Veterinary Science, Neston, United Kingdom

NEIL TOWNSEND, MSc, BVSc, Cert ES (Soft Tissue), MRCVS
Diplomate, European College of Surgery; Diplomate, European College of Veterinary Dentistry (Equine); Three Counties Equine Hospital, Tewksbury, Gloucestershire, United Kingdom

PAUL RENÉ VAN WEEREN, DVM, PhD
Diplomate, European College of Veterinary Surgeons; Department of Equine Sciences, Faculty of Veterinary Medicine, Utrecht University, Utrecht, The Netherlands

Contents

> Gerontology has become increasingly important in equine veterinary med-
> icine, with aged animals representing a significant proportion of the equine
> population. Horses are defined as geriatric or aged from age 15 years on-
> wards but can have a life span of more than 40 years. Despite a high level
> of owner concern for the well-being of their geriatric animal, provision of pre-
> ventive health care may be suboptimal. Owners seem to under-recognize
> some of the most prevalent diseases identified in geriatric horses. This re-
> view focuses on the demographic characteristics of the equine geriatric
> population and management and preventive care practices of older horses.

> Improved recognition of equine geriatric conditions has resulted in a surge
> in our aged population with a concurrent escalation of many age-related
> dental pathologies. Prevention of these disorder is the ultimate aim but
> early identification and appropriate management can increase an animal's
> oral comfort and maximise its masticatory ability. There is only a finite
> amount of tooth available for eruption in the horse and therefore as the
> teeth become worn and less efficient as a grinding unit, dietary modifica-
> tion becomes a paramount consideration to accommodate this. Geriatric
> animals have differing requirements for restraint and sedation with treat-
> ment of coexisting disorders also an important requirement.

> Musculoskeletal disorders are the most prevalent health problem in aging
> horses. They are not life threatening, but are painful and an important welfare
> issue. Chronic joint disease (osteoarthritis) and chronic laminitis are the most
> prevalent. Treating osteoarthritis in the elderly horse is similar to treating per-
> formance horses, but aims at providing a stable situation with optimal com-
> fort. Immediate medical treatment of flare-ups, long-term pain management,
> and adaptation of exercise and living conditions are the mainstays of treat-
> ment. Laminitis in the geriatric horse is related often to pituitary pars interme-
> dia dysfunction, which may be treated with additional pergolide.

> Ocular abnormalities are a common finding in aged horses. Although these
> seldom cause overt visual deficits detected by their owners, they can be a

source of chronic or acute discomfort so early detection, and treatment when available, is essential. Some of these abnormalities are specific to old horses, whereas others are a result of ongoing disease or inflammation that started earlier in life but that becomes more evident when the damage sustained to the eye is advanced. If vision is significantly affected, consideration of human safety and animal welfare is paramount.

Few skin diseases specifically or exclusively affect older horses and donkeys. Hypertrichosis (hirsutism) associated with pituitary pars intermedia dysfunction is probably the most recognized and best understood exception and is the most common age-related skin condition in equids. Many other conditions are known to be more serious in older horses. Horses affected with immune-compromising conditions can be more severely affected by infectious diseases of the skin or heavy and pathologically significant parasitism. Neoplasia of the skin is probably more prevalent and worse in older horses, although many of the more serious skin tumors develop initially at a younger age.

 Video content accompanies this article at http://www.vetequine. theclinics.com.

Respiratory and cardiac diseases are common in older horses. Advancing age is a specific risk factor for cardiac murmurs and these are more likely in males and small horses. Airway inflammation is the most common respiratory diagnosis. Recurrent airway obstruction can lead to irreversible structural change and bronchiectasis; with chronic hypoxia, right heart dysfunction and failure can develop. Valvular heart disease most often affects the aortic and/or the mitral valve. Management of comorbidity is an essential element of the therapeutic approach to cardiac and respiratory disease in older equids.

Aging horses may be at particular risk of endocrine disease. Two major equine endocrinopathies, pituitary pars intermedia dysfunction and equine metabolic syndrome, are commonly encountered in an aging population and may present with several recognizable signs, including laminitis. Investigation, treatment, and management of these diseases are discussed. Additionally, aging may be associated with development of rarer endocrinopathic problems, often associated with neoplasia, including diabetes mellitus and other confounders of glucose homeostasis, as well as thyroid, parathyroid, and adrenal diseases. Brief details of the recognition and management of these conditions are presented.

nonspecific chronic diseases. The decision to euthanize is difficult, so the advice of the veterinarian and QoL are important. This article focuses on the human–horse bond, assessment of QoL, reasons for euthanasia, and owner experiences of mortality.

VETERINARY CLINICS OF NORTH AMERICA: EQUINE PRACTICE

THE CLINICS ARE NOW AVAILABLE ONLINE!
Access your subscription at:
www.theclinics.com

Preface

Geriatric Medicine: Aged Horse Health, Management, and Welfare

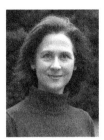

Catherine M. McGowan, BVSc, MACVS, DEIM,
DipECEIM, PhD, FHEA, MRCVS
Editor

It is with great pleasure that I introduce the 2016 version of Geriatric Medicine, which follows now 14 years after the excellent issue edited by Jennifer MacLeay in 2002. Although "Geriatric Medicine" implies a focus on disease diagnosis and management, this issue, like its predecessor, retains a focus on management and preventive care, successful aging, and quality of life, which are important aspects of aged horse care.

This issue has also benefited from a growing body of work in the veterinary literature that has taken place since 2002. In particular, the excellent epidemiology research, PhD theses, and subsequent publications by Dr Thomas McGowan and Dr Joanne Ireland on aged and geriatric horse health and welfare, respectively. In the first review, Dr Ireland introduces and discusses that work and the key findings, including the mismatch between a very apparent owner concern for their aged horses and their welfare, and their ability to recognize some of the most prevalent diseases.

The reviews involving the body systems in this issue reflect the highly prevalent conditions seen in both these studies: despite Dr McGowan's data coming from Australian horses and Dr Ireland's from UK horses, both studies had remarkable similarities, for example, in the prevalence and ranked frequency of the most important conditions seen in aged horses, notably dental and musculoskeletal diseases, integumentary and ophthalmological disorders, and cardiac, respiratory, and endocrine diseases. It is for this reason that this issue focuses on these body systems, with the valuable contributions from leading clinical specialists and researchers in these fields.

Another key finding was suboptimal preventive health care for some horses as they aged, but in particular, following retirement. This was despite owners clearly indicating their interest in maximizing their horse's health, welfare, and quality of life. In some

Vet Clin Equine 32 (2016) xi–xii
http://dx.doi.org/10.1016/j.cveq.2016.06.001
0749-0739/16/$ – see front matter © 2016 Published by Elsevier Inc.

cases, this was due to a lack of understanding; for example, owners assuming the cessation of travel or competition meant vaccination was no longer required. This issue contains reviews of exercise, immunology, and nutrition of aged horses from leading researchers in these areas.

I would like to thank all of the authors for their contributions to this vitally important area of equine practice. I hope readers will benefit from the valuable knowledge shared by these authors, pass the information on to their clients, and incorporate it into their daily clinical work for the benefit of all aged horses and their owners.

Catherine M. McGowan, BVSc, MACVS, DEIM, DipECEIM, PhD, FHEA, MRCVS
Faculty of Health and Life Sciences
University of Liverpool
Leahurst Campus
Wirral CH64 7TE, UK

E-mail address:
c.m.mcgowan@liverpool.ac.uk

Demographics, Management, Preventive Health Care and Disease in Aged Horses

Joanne L. Ireland, BVMS, PhD, Cert AVP(EM), MRCVS

KEYWORDS

- Demographic • Disease prevalence • Equine • Geriatric • Health care • Incidence
- Mortality

KEY POINTS

- Geriatric animals (aged ≥15 years) comprise up to one-third of the equine population.
- Management practices for geriatric horses, including exercise and diet, differ from those undertaken for the general equine population.
- Although geriatric horses may have a requirement for increased preventive health care, provision of several important preventive measures decreases with advancing horse age.
- Dental, musculoskeletal, endocrine, respiratory, and cardiovascular disorders are highly prevalent in geriatric horses.
- Owners may not be aware of the significance of clinical signs observed in their aged horse and seem to under-recognize some of the most prevalent diseases.

IMPORTANCE OF EQUINE GERIATRIC MEDICINE

Geriatric medicine involves knowledge of the diseases that are more common in aged patients and knowledge of how common diseases differ in their presentation in old age.[1] Geriatric medicine is a long-established specialty in human medicine, with the first medical textbook on aging published in the late 1800s. Geriatric medicine has also become increasingly important in equine veterinary medicine, with aged animals representing a growing proportion of referral hospital admissions.[2,3]

The fundamental role of the horse has changed over the past century, from use in agriculture and other industries to predominantly serving a role in the leisure industry[4] and, for some owners, toward that of a companion animal. Duration of ownership is often much longer for geriatric horses (10–14 years)[5–8] compared with younger horses

Disclosure Statement: The author has nothing to disclose.
Epidemiology and Disease Surveillance, Centre for Preventive Medicine, Animal Health Trust, Lanwades Park, Kentford, Newmarket, Suffolk CB8 7UU, UK
E-mail address: jo.ireland@aht.org.uk

Vet Clin Equine 32 (2016) 195–214
http://dx.doi.org/10.1016/j.cveq.2016.04.001
0749-0739/16/$ – see front matter © 2016 Elsevier Inc. All rights reserved.

(5–6 years),[6,9,10] which may enhance the owner-pet bond and subsequently influence owners' decision to seek and finance veterinary treatment.[11]

DEFINING THE GERIATRIC HORSE

The term, *geriatric*, first used in human medicine in the early 1900s, describes the life stage characterized by progressive decline in physical condition, organ function, and immunity.[12] The age at which a horse is defined as geriatric or aged seems to have changed over the past several decades and remains a subject for debate. The age at which an individual is categorized as geriatric can be defined in different ways, including chronologic age, demographic age, and physiologic or functional age.[13] In using these various definitions, research studies investigating health and disease in aged horses have selected different chronologic ages (most frequently from 15 to 20 years and over) as the inclusion criterion for their study populations, which can make direct comparison of their results more difficult.

Several terms are used to describe people considered old, but there is an increasing awareness that the terms used should acknowledge the tremendous diversity inherent in a group of people whose ages can span a range of 40 or more years.[14] Because horses may be defined as geriatric from age 15 onwards, but can have a life span of more than 40 years, adopting a categorical classification to describe aged animals based on terminology used in human geriatrics may be beneficial in accounting for some of the wide individual variations in rates of aging between horses. Categorization of all equids greater than 20 years of age as geriatric may fail to differentiate significant physiologic differences within this group.[6] Based on available survivorship data for the equine population, using a definition by demographic age, horses and ponies aged greater than or equal to 15 years are defined as old whereas those aged greater than or equal to 30 years are defined as very old.[8,15–19]

The average life expectancy within the general equine population has been reported as 19 years.[20] Although there are reports of horses surviving into their 50s, it seems the life span of the horse is reached at approximately 45 years, based on the oldest animals included in various research studies.[2,8,17,18]

DEMOGRAPHICS OF THE EQUINE GERIATRIC POPULATION

Population aging is an important feature of the human population, with the very old age category (those aged ≥85 years) the fastest growing section,[21] and demographers expect to see this high growth of the oldest old group continue.[14] In comparison to the human population, there is limited demographic information regarding the equine population. A survey in the United Kingdom found 25% of horses were aged greater than 15 years, with 70% survival of the population at 15 years and less than 50% survival of the population over 20 years.[15] A subsequent study, including a larger geographic area, reported that 28% of the UK equine population were greater than or equal to 15 years old.[16] More recently, 29.5% of horses and ponies in the UK were reported to be aged greater than or equal to 15 years, with a decline in numbers within the population after the age of 15 years, and only 2.2% aged greater than 30 years.[8] In Australia, McGowan and colleagues[17] found that 33.7% of horses were aged greater than or equal to 15 years, whereas another large owner questionnaire survey, also conducted in Australia, found 18.9% of horses were aged greater than or equal to 16 years, with 7.7% greater than 20 years of age.[18] Data from the National Animal Health Monitoring System in the United States, comprising information from equestrian operations with greater than or equal to 5 resident equids, showed 7.6% of the equine population were aged greater than or equal to 20 years and only

0.7% aged greater than or equal to 30 years.[22] An on-line survey, including multiple countries (predominantly in Europe and North America and Canada), reported that 28% of horses owned by respondents were aged greater than or equal to 16 years.[19]

With increasing age, pony breeds become over-represented within the geriatric population.[2,5,22–25] Breed distribution varies widely, however, between different countries, making direct comparisons difficult and precluding assessment of increased longevity in particular breeds. For example, compared with the UK equine population,[9,15] there is a much lower proportion of pony breeds in the United States[6,22,25,26] and differences in demographic characteristics are likely to have an effect on the management and health conditions in these different populations. The difference in the proportion of pony breeds in equine populations between different countries may also go some way to explaining the observed differences in age distribution.

In the human population, women seem to have increased life expectancy and there is an increased proportion of women compared with men in the geriatric population.[14,21] This effect does not seem evident in the equine population, where male horses are over-represented.[6,8,17,25,27] The predominance of male horses in geriatric equine populations, however, does not seem to differ from that of the general population,[6,9,10,25] although the proportion of entire male horses tends to be greater in nongeriatric populations, reflecting that studies of the general equine population include colts prior to castration.

MANAGEMENT OF THE GERIATRIC HORSE

Management practices, including exercise and nutrition, may affect equine health and welfare. Furthermore, specific husbandry measures may be required for the successful management of certain disease conditions. There is limited published information, however, regarding management practices, particularly for the geriatric section of the equine population. Although a high level of owner management has been reported for geriatric horses,[6,8,17] there is some evidence to suggest that management practices may be reduced once animals are retired.[17]

Stable Management and Housing

Horses are kept on a wide variety of types of premises, and the attributes of different premises may have significant effects on management practices and risk factors for disease. A vast majority of geriatric horses have regular turnout to grazing for at least part of the year, with few animals stabled continuously[6,8,17]; however, duration of field turnout varies considerably between seasons.[8] Although there may be differences between countries, with a greater proportion of horses kept predominantly indoors in stalls in the United States, general stable management of geriatric horses seems little different compared with that reported for younger animals.[6]

Feeding and Nutrition

In addition to grazing, almost all geriatric horses are fed some form of preserved forage feed, most frequently hay[6,17,19] or haylage.[8] Dental disease in the geriatric horse may reduce their ability to effectively masticate long-fiber forage feeds, and hay replacers are more commonly fed to older horses[6,8] and those with dental disease or displaying quidding or difficulty eating.[8]

There has been an increase in availability of veteran types of feeds in recent years, with an extensive range of commercial veteran/senior diets and complete mash feeds specifically marketed for use in older horses. Many of these geriatric feed products were developed based on early research findings that suggested older horses had reduced apparent digestion of crude protein, phosphorus, and fiber compared with younger horses fed the same diet.[28] Subsequent research demonstrated, however, that the apparent reduction in digestive efficiency with age, which was attributed to decreased digestive or absorptive processes in the large intestine, was less substantial than previously reported and the investigators hypothesized that the physiologic changes observed in their earlier work may have been secondary to parasite damage.[29–31] A more recent study, randomly assigning horses to receive 1 of 3 different diets, found no differences in the digestibility/apparent digestibility of energy, neutral detergent fiber, crude protein, fat, calcium, or phosphorus between adult horses (aged 5–12 years) and geriatric horses (aged 19–28 years).[32]

Senior diets remain popular with horse owners and are frequently used in older horses.[6,8,19] Increasing horse age has been associated with dietary changes,[8,17,27] with 40% of owners reporting making major changes to their horses' diet as they had aged.[8] Weight loss is frequently reported by owners of geriatric horses,[27,33,34] considered the most important health issue in geriatric horses,[33] and seems a major motivating factor in implementing dietary changes.[19] Obesity, however, is more prevalent in aged horses.[6,34,35] Both weight loss and obesity have a significant effect on morbidity and mortality in the geriatric equine population and represent different challenges in the nutritional management of aged horses.

Exercise

Many geriatric horses continue to participate in regular athletic activity, encompassing a similar range of disciplines reported for their younger counterparts.[6,8,17] With increasing age, horses are more likely to be retired.[5,6,8,17] Although a majority of geriatric horses are still in ridden exercise, the duration and intensity of exercise decrease with increasing age.[8,17]

PREVENTIVE HEALTH CARE FOR THE AGED HORSE

There is limited published information regarding the role of routine health care in equine geriatric medicine; therefore, recommendations are largely extrapolated from those for younger animals. Veterinary assessments play an important role in any preventive health care program; however, a significant proportion of geriatric horses do not receive regular routine veterinary visits,[17] and nonemergency veterinary attention decreases with increasing age[34] and retirement.[17,34]

Vaccination

Although specific equine vaccination recommendations vary between different countries, vaccinations against tetanus and equine influenza are consistently the most frequently administered. Aged horses remain susceptible to infection with equine influenza virus despite the presence of circulating antibodies; however, vaccination provided protection against clinical disease and reduced virus shedding.[36]

One UK study found that a higher proportion of geriatric horses (30%) were never vaccinated compared with young horses (14%) and that the frequency of vaccination was reduced in older horses.[20] More recently, the proportion of geriatric horses vaccinated against tetanus and equine influenza[34] was comparable to the proportion of vaccinated animals in the general equine population.[37] Regular vaccination for either disease was reduced, however, with both increasing age and retirement.[34] Although increasing horse age was an infrequent reason for nonvaccination, animals not participating in competition or travelling from their farm area were major factors reported by Finnish owners for not vaccinating horses of all ages.[38] The most frequent reason for failure to maintain regular vaccinations reported by owners was a perceived reduction in risk of disease, with a perception that older horses had lasting immunity from prior vaccination and were less likely to travel off their home premises or to mix with other horses.[39] For every year's increase in age, geriatric horses had a 40% decreased likelihood of regular tetanus vaccination.[17] Communicating the importance of maintaining appropriate vaccination schedules to both veterinary surgeons and horse owners may increase the practice of this particularly important preventive health care measure, with the additional benefit of ensuring that geriatric horses are attended by a veterinary surgeon on an annual basis, which may provide an opportunity for early disease detection.

Dental Prophylaxis

Although a majority of geriatric horses receive some degree of regular dental prophylaxis,[34] 1 study reported that a greater proportion of aged horses did not receive annual dental care compared with younger horses (11% and 2%, respectively).[6] Despite owners ranking teeth and dental care as the third most important health issue in geriatric horses and 18% reporting it as a major health concern,[33] 33% of horses had not received any dental care within the previous 12 months.[17] In addition to individual horse factors and dietary considerations, the frequency and standards of dental prophylaxis are likely to have some effect on the development and subsequent management of dental disease in the geriatric horse.

Anthelmintic Administration

The intensity of naturally occurring *Anoplocephala perfoliata* infection, determined by IgG antibody response, increases in geriatric horses.[23,40] Conversely, a small study found no correlation between increasing age and fecal strongyle egg counts prior to, or 12 weeks after, ivermectin administration,[41] and another study found that a majority of horses aged greater than or equal to 30 years had low fecal worm egg counts.[23] A more recent study, however, has identified significantly higher fecal strongyle egg counts in geriatric horses (aged 20–33 years) compared with adult horses (aged 5–15 years).[42]

As a result of increasing resistance to commonly used anthelmintics, recommendations regarding worming strategies have changed in recent years; therefore, simply considering total number of anthelmintic treatments per year or frequency of administration is unlikely sufficient in assessing the adequacy of anthelmintic use in geriatric horses. Although the majority of geriatric horses are regularly administered anthelmintic products,[6,17,34] older animals may receive less frequent parasite control.[6,17,20]

Farrier Care

Hoof problems, including imbalances, sand cracks, and issues related to horn quality, are highly prevalent in geriatric horses[35] and may be influenced by degenerative changes, concurrent disease, and nutritional factors.[43] In the United Kingdom, recommendations by the National Equine Welfare Council indicate that hooves should be checked by a registered farrier every 4 to 8 weeks.[44] Although some studies have reported that a vast majority of geriatric horses receive regular hoof care,[6,17] others have found that geriatric horses receive less frequent farrier visits compared with younger horses.[20,34] Reduced frequency of routine hoof care in geriatric horses may not only exacerbate hoof problems but also influence the development or progression of musculoskeletal disorders.

SIGNS OF AGING

When assessing geriatric health and disease, it is important to recognize and distinguish between benign signs of aging, age-related physiologic changes that predispose to disease, and clinical signs of disease associated with aging. In early human geriatric medicine, Perlman[45] suggested that normal aging could be distinguished from chronic degenerative conditions. Accurately making this distinction in aging horses, however, can be difficult for both owners and veterinary surgeons. Owners of geriatric horses report observing signs that they perceived as signs of aging at 19 to 23 years of age.[6,27,34]

Senescence is defined as the condition or process of deterioration with age, and commonly considered benign signs of senescence in horses include increasing grey hairs, particularly around the eyes and muzzle; drooping of the lower lip; loss of muscle tone; and deepening of the hollows above the eyes.[46] Other changes frequently described as signs of aging, such as alternations in hair coat, decreased feed efficiency,[47] musculoskeletal stiffness or reduced joint flexibility, and exercise intolerance/fatigue,[27] are likely to represent clinical signs of disease.

DISEASES OF AGED HORSES

In human geriatric medicine, chronic illness is responsible for a majority of deaths and accounts for more than 87% of health problems in people aged greater than or equal to 60 years.[48] Elderly animals seldom have a single disease,[12] and factors influencing the rate of development of both normal aging and chronic diseases are often identical.[49]

Although owner-reported disease prevalence increases with increasing horse age,[17,18,34] veterinary examination of a small group of geriatric horses considered by their owners as healthy revealed several prevalent health conditions.[5] This suggests owners may under-recognize or under-report disease in geriatric horses; therefore, owner-reported information may not provide accurate prevalence estimates for some common disorders.

Although increasing age has been reported as a risk factor for an array of different conditions, it has only been within the past 15 years that research studies have sought to estimate the prevalence of diseases affecting geriatric horses (**Table 1**). As may be expected, acute conditions, such as colic, are reported more frequently in referral hospital populations, whereas the prevalence of chronic conditions is considerably higher in field-based studies (see **Table 1**).

Musculoskeletal Disorders and Lameness

It is possible that age-related changes in the musculoskeletal system contribute to the development of orthopedic disease in geriatric horses by increasing the effects of other risk factors, including abnormal biomechanics, joint injury, genetics, and obesity.[50] Musculoskeletal disorders are a major reason for euthanasia in horses of all ages[51–54] and the most frequent cause of mortality in geriatric horses.[55] At postmortem examination of geriatric horses, the musculoskeletal system was the second most frequently affected body system,[24] and retrospective analysis of insurance claims for mortality found that horses greater than 15 years of age were significantly more likely to have a nontraumatic cause of fatal locomotor disease compared with younger animals.[56] Lameness was the second most common reason overall for referral in one study,[2] but conversely, older horses were significantly less likely than younger animals to be presented for musculoskeletal disorders in another referral

Table 1
Prevalence estimates of disease in geriatric horses and ponies based on owner-reported data or veterinary clinical examination findings

	Owner-Reported Disease Prevalence					Disease Prevalence Observed at Veterinary Clinical Examination				
Study Reference	Brosnahan & Paradis,[6] 2003	McGowan et al,[33] 2010	Ireland et al,[34] 2011	Ireland et al,[23] 2011	Chandler & Mellor,[5] 2001	Brosnahan & Paradis,[2] 2003	McGowan,[7] 2009, and McGowan et al,[93] 2013	Ireland et al,[35] 2012	Ireland et al,[23] 2011	Silva & Furr,[25] 2013
Country	USA	Australia	UK	UK	UK	USA	Australia	UK	UK	USA
Study design	Cross-sectional –questionnaire survey	Cross-sectional study – postal questionnaire survey	Cross-sectional study – postal questionnaire survey	Cross-sectional study – postal questionnaire survey	Cross-sectional pilot study	Retrospective review of clinical records	Cross-sectional study	Cross-sectional study	Cross-sectional study	Retrospective review of clinical records
Selection of study population	Veterinary-registered horse owners plus owners attending geriatric horse lectures	Members of a regional equestrian group	Veterinary-registered horse owners	Veterinary-registered horse owners	Horses presented to the ambulatory service of a veterinary medical teaching hospital for a "free health check"	Horses presented to a veterinary medical teaching hospital	Subset of horses included in study 33 selected by convenience sampling	Subset of horses included in study 34 selected by systematic random sampling	All respondents in study 23 invited to participate	Horses presented to a referral hospital
Number of horses/ponies	165	974	918	87	23	467	339	200	69	345
Age inclusion criterion	≥20 y	≥15 y	≥15 y	≥30 y	Not stated	≥20 y	≥15 y	≥15 y	≥30 y	≥20 y
Age of study population	Mean 26.5 y (range 20–44 y)	Median 20.7 y (range 15–44 y)	Median 20 y (interquartile range 17–24 y)	Median 31.2 y (range 30–45 y)	Median 26.5 y	Median 24 y (range 20–45 y)	Mean 20.5 y (95% CI, 20.0–21.1 y)	Median 20 y (interquartile range 17–25 y)	—	Mean 23.9 y (range 20–36 y)

(continued on next page)

Table 1
(continued)

Study Reference	Owner-Reported Disease Prevalence				Disease Prevalence Observed at Veterinary Clinical Examination					
	Brosnahan & Paradis,[6] 2003	McGowan et al,[33] 2010	Ireland et al,[34] 2011	Ireland et al,[23] 2011	Chandler & Mellor,[5] 2001	Brosnahan & Paradis,[2] 2003	McGowan,[7] 2009, and McGowan et al,[93] 2013	Ireland et al,[35] 2012	Ireland et al,[23] 2011	Silva & Furr,[25] 2013
Disease prevalence estimated based on	Timeframe not stated	Period prevalence of disease within previous 12 mo* or point prevalence of owner-reported current condition#	Period prevalence of disease within previous 12 mo* or point prevalence of owner-reported current condition#	Period prevalence of disease within previous 12 mo* or point prevalence of owner-reported current condition#	Apparent prevalence at single veterinary examination	Apparent prevalence based on hospital records (549 admissions for 467 horses)	Apparent prevalence at single veterinary examination	Apparent prevalence at single veterinary examination	Apparent prevalence at single veterinary examination	Apparent prevalence based on hospital records
Lameness (excluding laminitis)	NR (geriatric horses more likely than animals aged <20 y to have history of lameness [P<.001])	28.0%* (95% CI, 25.4%–30.8%) 7.4%# (95% CI, 5.8%–9.0%)	24.2%* (95% CI, 21.4%–27.0%)	18.4%* (95% CI, 10.2%–26.5%)	NR	17.1% (95% CI, 13.7%–20.5%)	50.4% (95% CI, 45.2%–55.7%)	50.5% (95% CI, 43.4%–57.6%)	77.3% (95% CI, 67.2%–87.4%)	19.8% (95% CI, 15.6%–24.0%)

Laminitis (current and/or historical)	NR	4.8%* (95% CI, 3.5%–6.1%) 2.0%# (95% CI, 1.1%–2.9%)	6.8%* (95% CI, 5.1%–8.4%) 3.3%# (95% CI, 2.1%–4.4%)	6.9%* (95% CI, 1.6%–12.2%)	NR	6.4% (95% CI, 4.2%–8.6%)	NR	6.2% (95% CI, 3.7%–8.8%) had owner-reported history of laminitis within preceding 12 mo[93]	NR	1.0% (95% CI, 0–2.4%) had acute laminitis at time of examination 7.5% Had owner-reported history of laminitis within preceding 12 mo[96]	NR	1.7% (95% CI, 0.3%–3.1%)
Dental disorders	10.4% (95% CI, 5.7%–15.1%)	10.0%* (95% CI, 8.1%–11.9%)	19.1%* (95% CI, 16.5%–21.6%)	44.8%# (95% CI, 34.4%–55.3%)	47.8% (95% CI, 27.4%–68.2%)	7.8% (95% CI, 5.5%–10.4%) * dental problems were presenting complaint for only 8.1% of animals with dental disease	96.4% (95% CI, 94.3%–98.4%)	95.4% (95% CI, 92.3%–98.5%)	100% (95% CI, 94.0%–100%)	0.9% (95% CI, 0–1.8%)
Colic	NR (geriatric horses more likely than animals aged <20 y to have history of colic (P = .01))	7.7% (95% CI, 6.0%–9.4%)	8.7%* (95% CI, 6.9%–10.5%)	6.9%* (95% CI, 1.6%–12.2%)	0 (95% CI, 0–0.14%)	38.8% (95% CI, 34.3%–43.1%)	0 (95% CI, 0–0.01%)	0 (95% CI, 0–0.02%)	0 (95% CI, 0–6.0%)	38.8% (95% CI, 33.7%–44.0%)

(continued on next page)

Table 1
(continued)

Study Reference	Owner-Reported Disease Prevalence				Disease Prevalence Observed at Veterinary Clinical Examination					
	Brosnahan & Paradis,[6] 2003	McGowan et al,[33] 2010	Ireland et al,[34] 2011	Ireland et al,[23] 2011	Chandler & Mellor,[5] 2001	Brosnahan & Paradis,[2] 2003	McGowan,[7] 2009, and McGowan et al,[93] 2013	Ireland et al,[35] 2012	Ireland et al,[23] 2011	Silva & Furr,[25] 2013
Respiratory disorders	NR	18.7%* (95% CI, 16.2%–21.1%)	7.4%* (95% CI, 5.7%–9.1%)	8.0%* (95% CI, 2.3%–13.8%)	39.1% (95% CI, 19.2%–59.1%)	15.6% (95% CI, 12.3%–18.9%)	21.0% (95% CI, 16.7%–25.3%)	22.0% (95% CI, 16.3%–27.7%)	31.9% (95% CI, 20.9%–42.9%)	5.5% (95% CI, 3.1%–7.9%)
Cardiovascular disorders	NR	0.4%# (95% CI, 0–0.8%)	0.5%# (95% CI, 0.06%–1.0%)	NR	60.9% (95% CI, 40.9%–80.8%)	7.1% (95% CI, 4.7%–9.4%)	43.2% (95% CI, 38.0%–48.4%)	24.5% (95% CI, 18.5%–30.5%)	43.5% (95% CI, 31.8%–55.1%)	2.9% (95% CI, 1.1%–4.7%)
Dermatologic disorders	NR	21.0%* (95% CI, 18.4%–23.6%)	7.1%* (95% CI, 5.4%–8.7%)	6.9%* (95% CI, 1.6%–12.2%)	65.2% (95% CI, 45.8%–84.7%)	6.2% (95% CI, 4.0%–8.4%)	40.1% (95% CI, 34.9%–45.2%)	71.0% (95% CI, 64.7%–77.3%)	NR	7.3% (95% CI, 4.5%–10.0%)
Hypertrichosis/hair coat abnormalities	30.1% (95% CI, 23.0%–37.15%)	16.8%* (95% CI, 14.5%–19.1%)	12.5%* (95% CI, 10.4%–14.7%)	37.9%* (95% CI, 27.7%–48.1%)	NR	NR	13.8% (95% CI, 10.2%–17.5%)	22.0% (95% CI, 16.3%–27.7%)	44.9% (95% CI, 33.2%–56.7%)	NR
PPID	8.0% (95% CI, 3.8%–12.1%)	1.6%# (95% CI, 0.8%–2.4%)	3.3%# (95% CI, 2.1%–4.4%)	12.6%# (95% CI, 5.7–19.6%)	39.1% (95% CI, 19.2%–59.1%)	9.8% (95% CI, 7.1%–12.6%)	21.2% (95% CI, 16.9%–26.1%)[93]	NR	NR	NR (0.3%, n = 1, presented for unspecified endocrine disease)
Owner-reported weight loss/poor condition or BCS <2/5 on clinical examination	4.2% (95% CI, 1.2%–7.3%)	16.9%* (95% CI, 14.5%–19.3%)	Weight loss 16.8%* (95% CI, 14.4%–19.2%) Underweight 8.2%# (95% CI, 6.4%–9.9%)	Weight loss 40.2%* (95% CI, 29.9%–50.5%) Underweight 23.2%# (95% CI, 13.2%–33.1%)	34.8% (95% CI, 15.3%–54.2%)	NR	2.1% (95% CI, 0.5%–3.6%)	4.5% (95% CI, 1.6%–7.4%)	15.9% (95% CI, 7.3%–24.6%)	NR

Owner-reported overweight/ obesity or BCS ≥3.5/5 on clinical examination BCS	28.5% (95% CI, 21.6%–35.4%)	NR	10.5%# (95% CI, 8.5%–12.4%)	2.9%# (95% CI, 0–6.9%)	NR	NR	29.7% (95% CI, 24.9%–34.5%)	26.0% (95% CI, 19.9%–32.1%)	10.1% (95% CI, 3.0%–17.3%) / NR
Ocular disorders	NR	3.3%# (95% CI, 2.3%–4.3%)	3.5%* (95% CI, 2.3%–4.7%)	5.7%* (95% CI, 0.8%–10.6%)	65.2% (95% CI, 45.8%–84.7%)	10.7% (95% CI, 7.9%–13.5%)	87.8% (95% CI, 84.2%–91.3%)	94.0% (95% CI, 90.1%–97.3%)	100% (95% CI, 94.7%–100%) / NR
Neoplasia (predominantly cutaneous)	NR (geriatric horses more likely than animals aged <20 y to have history of neoplasia (P = .04))	4.2%# (95% CI, 2.9%–5.4%)	2.2%# (95% CI, 1.2%–3.1%)	1.1%# (95% CI, 0–3.4%)	NR	10.1% (95% CI, 7.3%–12.8%)	10.7% (95% CI, 7.4%–13.9%)	15.5% (95% CI, 10.5%–20.5%) / NR	9.6% (95% CI, 6.5%–12.7%)
Reproductive disorders	NR	0.7%# (95% CI, 0.2%–1.2%)	0.8%* (95% CI, 0.2%–1.3%)	NR	NR	5.8% (95% CI, 3.7%–7.9%)	NR	NR	NR
Neurologic disorders	NR	0.8%# (95% CI, 0.2%–1.4%)	0.8%# (95% CI, 0.2%–1.3%)	1.1%* (95% CI, 0–3.4%)	NR	4.5% (95% CI, 2.6%–6.4%)	10.4% (95% CI, 7.2%–13.6%)	NR	1.7% (95% CI, 0.4%–3.1%)
Urinary tract disorders	NR	3.7%* (95% CI, 2.5%–4.9%)	0.3%* (95% CI, 0–0.7%)	1.1%* (95% CI, 0–3.4%)	NR	2.8% (95% CI, 1.3%–4.3%)	0 (95% CI, 0–0.01%)	0 (95% CI, 0–0.02%)	5.5% (95% CI, 3.1%–7.9%)
Hemolymphatic disorders	NR	0 (95% CI, 0–0.4%)	0.4%* (95% CI, 0.1–0.9%)	NR	NR	1.9% (95% CI, 0.7%–3.2%)	0 (95% CI, 0–0.01%)	0 (95% CI, 0–0.02%)	1.4% (95% CI, 0.2–2.7%)

Asymptotic 95% CIs (or Wilson score intervals for small sample sizes) were calculated where not reported in the original publication. Figures in italic font indicate unpublished data – data were presented combined with other results in publications[23,34,35] (Jo Ireland, unpublished data, 2010).

Abbreviation: NR, not reported.

* Period prevalence of disease within previous 12 months.

Point prevalence of owner-reported current condition.

hospital population.[25] Based on both owner-reported and veterinary data, osteoarthritis is the most prevalent musculoskeletal condition in geriatric horses.[2,25,33,34]

Lameness is considered an important health problem by horse owners,[57,58] yet the owner-reported prevalence of musculoskeletal disease is considerably lower than the prevalence of associated clinical signs.[33,34] This indicates that lameness is under-recognized or considered less important by owners of geriatric animals, particularly where the horse is retired from ridden exercise.[2] Agreement between experienced equine veterinary surgeons evaluating lameness in horses is low, suggesting that subjective assessment of horses with mild lameness is not reliable,[59] implying that mild–moderate lameness may be difficult for owners to detect, especially in retired horses.

Laminitis

Laminitis was one of the most frequent specific diagnoses in geriatric horses presenting to a referral hospital, accounting for 6% of cases overall and 37.5% of cases examined due to lameness.[2] Increasing age has been associated with an increased risk of both acute[60] and chronic laminitis.[60-62] The increased risk of laminitis in older horses is often attributed to pituitary pars intermedia dysfunction (PPID). Studies have reported concurrent and/or historical laminitis in 24% to 82% of horses diagnosed with PPID.[2,63-66]

Dental Disease

Dental disease is the main oral disorder of horses and is most commonly caused by disorders of wear, as a result of the horse's masticatory action. There is evidence to suggest that owners under-recognize dental disease or may fail to attribute associated clinical signs to a dental disorder. Owner-reported prevalence of clinical signs of dental disease, such as dysmastication (quidding or difficulty eating), is considerably higher than the owner-reported prevalence of dental disorders.[6,33,34]

The most prevalent dental disorders in geriatric horses include tooth loss, diastemata, periodontal disease, and abnormalities of wear, such as focal overgrowths, wave mouth, shear mouth, and smooth mouth,[7,23,35,67] with a considerable proportion of affected animals having moderate to severe dental disease.[7] Despite the high prevalence of dental disorders in geriatric horses, the management of dental disease has been improved by increased knowledge of pathophysiology and treatment options, availability of advanced dental equipment, and increased availability of diets designed for horses with dysmastication.

Colic

Colic is the most common gastrointestinal tract abnormality seen in equine practice and is the most frequent reason for referral in horses greater than or equal to 20 years old[2,25] (see **Table 1**). There is limited published information regarding incidence of colic in the geriatric population; however, colic was the second most common reason for euthanasia in 1 study.[55] Causes of colic in geriatric horses differ compared with the most common causes reported in nongeriatric horses,[25,68] and higher prevalence of certain types of colic in aged horses has been reported.

Cecal impactions have been reported to occur with increasing frequency in older horses.[69,70] Dental disease and reduced frequency of dental treatment have been associated with an increased risk of colic,[71,72] and the increased risk of large colon impactions in geriatric horses has primarily been attributed to poor dentition.[2] Increasing age has also been associated with increased incidence of strangulating lipomas.[2,25,73-76] Among cases referred for colic, geriatric horses aged greater than or equal to 16 years were twice as likely to have a strangulating small intestinal lesion compared with nongeriatric adult horses (aged 4–15 years) and were significantly less likely to have a large colon lesion.[68]

Geriatric horses treated for colic had reduced short-term survival compared with mature horses.[68,77] Overall survival rate after surgical treatment of colic, however, was not significantly different, and only horses aged greater than or equal to 20 years had a lower survival rate after surgery.[68] Similarly, there was no consistent association between increasing age and mortality in a study of long-term survival of surgical colic cases.[78] The association between age and decreased survival appears after surgery for large intestinal disease but not for small intestinal disease.[79,80] Another study reported that survival after colic surgery was greater in very old horses (aged ≥30 years) compared with horses aged 20 to 29 years (61% and 53%, respectively).[2] Of 23 geriatric horses euthanized due to colic, none had received surgical treatment[55]; therefore, it is possible that surgical intervention is undertaken less frequently in geriatric horses and referral for surgery is more likely where cases are considered to have a favorable prognosis.[2]

Respiratory Disease

In a referral hospital population, the third most commonly affected body system in horses aged greater than or equal to 20 years was the respiratory system, accounting for 16% of all cases[2] (see **Table 1**). Although clinical signs of respiratory disease, such as coughing and nasal discharge, are frequently reported by owners of geriatric horses, the owner-reported prevalence of respiratory disease is considerably lower,[33,34,81] suggesting that respiratory disease is under-recognized or undiagnosed in a considerable proportion of aged animals.

Recurrent airway obstruction (RAO) is the most prevalent respiratory disease in geriatric horses. Within the general equine population in the UK, the prevalence of RAO, determined using a risk screening questionnaire, was reported as 14% with both increasing age and retirement identified as risk factors for the disease.[82] Using the same risk screening questionnaire, the prevalence of RAO in a geriatric population was estimated as 20.7%; however, the median age at which animals were diagnosed with RAO was 13 years and there was no increased risk of RAO with increasing age over 18 years.[83] Despite reporting clinical signs, 91% of owners of RAO-affected horses were satisfied with their current health status, implying some degree of acceptance by owners of even severe clinical signs.[84] Owner-reported coughing and nasal discharge were associated with veterinary clinical examination findings, arterial oxygen tensions, tracheal endoscopy mucus scores, and airway responsiveness determined by histamine challenge in RAO-affected horses.[84]

Cardiovascular Disease

In horses of any age, cardiac murmurs are commonly detected as an incidental finding because many valvular insufficiencies are clinically well tolerated[85] and progression to congestive heart failure is rare.[86] This may go some way to explaining the low owner-reported prevalence of cardiovascular disease, with cardiac disease reported in less than or equal to 0.5% of geriatric horses.[33,34] Although considerably greater than the owner-reported prevalence, cardiovascular disorders comprise a small proportion of geriatric cases in referral hospital populations[2,25] (see **Table 1**).

Increasing age has been identified as a significant risk factor associated with left-sided valvular regurgitation/insufficiencies (LSVRs), such as aortic and mitral insufficiency.[54,87] The prevalence of LSVRs increased with age, from 3.4% in horses aged less than 8 years to 13.5% in horses aged 15 to 23 years and 14.8% in horses greater than or equal to 24 years; however, there was no significant difference in the mortality of horses with and without LSVRs.[54] In a small group of geriatric horses with no owner-reported health problems, 60.9% had cardiac murmurs at veterinary examination, with 17.4% of these aged horses having cardiac murmurs of greater than or equal to grade 4.[5]

Pituitary Pars Intermedia Dysfunction

PPID is an age-related dopaminergic neurodegenerative disease affecting the pars intermedia of the pituitary gland.[88,89] The most frequently reported clinical signs of PPID include hypertrichosis (or abnormal hair coat shedding and other hair coat abnormalities, often referred to collectively as *hirsutism*), laminitis, epaxial muscle wastage, weight loss, and lethargy or depression.[90–92]

PPID is the most common endocrine disorder of older equines, reported as the most frequently diagnosed endocrine condition in geriatric horses aged greater than or equal to 20 years.[2] Published prevalence estimates vary widely, however, depending on type and sample population used in different studies. The prevalence of veterinary-diagnosed PPID, based on elevated basal corticotropin using seasonally adjusted reference ranges, was reported as 21.2% in a large study of horses aged greater than or equal to 15 years.[93]

The owner-reported prevalence of PPID in geriatric horses is considerably lower (≤8%)[6,33,34]; however, owners frequently report hair coat changes compatible with clinical signs of pituitary dysfunction, including hypertrichosis and incomplete shedding, in horses that have not been diagnosed with PPID.[6,33,34] Overt hypertrichosis is considered a highly specific indicator of PPID,[93,94] and owner-reported hair coat abnormalities are significantly associated with increasing horse age.[27,33,34] To date, only increasing age has been identified as a risk factor for PPID within the geriatric population.[93]

Ocular Disorders

Ophthalmic lesions are identified in a large proportion of geriatric horses (≥65%).[5,7,35,95] Degeneration of the vitreous, senile retinopathy, and cataracts are among the most common lesions identified,[7,35,95] with the prevalence of these lesions increasing with advancing age.[35,95] Despite the high prevalence of ocular lesions, few owners report visual disturbances[95,96] and those who did report visual deficits found these were worse in poor light.[95] Many geriatric horses may be retired or working at a reduced level; therefore, owners may be less likely to detect visual deficits. It is also possible that geriatric horses cope well with poor vision, and also that many of the common ophthalmic conditions of the aging horse are slowly progressive, allowing the animal to become accustomed to reduced vision.

Neoplasia

It seems commonly considered that horses have a low incidence of neoplasia,[51,97] with few tumors occurring exclusively in geriatric horses and ponies.[97] Neoplasia, however, was the most common specific diagnosis in geriatric animals in a referral hospital population.[25] In a large review of post-mortem examinations, neoplasia was common in geriatric horses and increased in prevalence with increasing age, representing the most common individual diagnosis in horses aged greater than or equal to 25 years.[24] Pituitary adenoma was the most prevalent neoplasia identified in this post-mortem study.[24] Nonfunctional pars intermedia adenomas have been described, however, in aged horses, showing no signs of endocrine disorders such as PPID.[98] Neoplasia, excluding PPID, was identified in 17% of horses aged greater than or equal to 20 years in a referral hospital population.[2]

Tumors affecting the skin are the most common form of equine neoplasia. Melanoma represented 10% of neoplasias in geriatric horses treated at a referral hospital.[2] Squamous cell carcinomas and melanomas are often diagnosed in middle age, with a mean age at diagnosis of approximately 11 years.[99] Squamous cell carcinomas were the most frequently diagnosed neoplasia in geriatric horses, comprising 38% of cases.[2] Thyroid adenomas were reported in 75% of horses greater than 20 years of age at post-mortem.[100] These nodular lesions were identified as C-cell adenomas and suspected to be nonfunctional and unlikely to lead to calcitonin hypersecretion-related diseases.[100]

The prevalence of abdominal lipomas increases with age, with a mean age of approximately 17 to 19 years.[74–76] Lymphomas are often found in younger animals and in 1 study approximately half of cases were aged less than or equal to 5 years.[101] For mediastinal lymphosarcoma, the mean age of cases has been reported as 10 to 12 years.[102,103] Lymphosarcoma, however, accounted for 9% of neoplasias in geriatric horses.[2]

SUMMARY

Geriatric horses and ponies represent a significant proportion of the equine population and are of great importance to their owners. Despite this level of concern, provision of preventive health care may be suboptimal and owners seem to under-recognize some of the most prevalent diseases identified in geriatric horses. Under-recognition of disease and insufficient knowledge regarding the significance of clinical signs may result in owners failing to seek appropriate veterinary attention for common health conditions in the geriatric horse, without which there may be reduced provision of effective treatment, compromised welfare, and increased risk of mortality. There is a clear requirement for improved targeted education of both horse owners and the veterinary profession, which would be a significant step towards achieving successful aging in the horse.

REFERENCES

1. Fillit HM, Rockwood K, Woodhouse K. Introduction: aging, frailty, and geriatric medicine. In: Fillit HM, Rockwood K, Woodhouse K, editors. Brocklehurst's textbook of geriatric medicine and gerontology. 7th edition. Philadelphia: Saunders Elsevier; 2010. p. 1–2.
2. Brosnahan MM, Paradis MR. Demographic and clinical characteristics of geriatric horses: 467 cases (1989-1999). J Am Vet Med Assoc 2003;223:93–8.
3. Traub-Dargatz JL, Long RE, Bertone JJ. What is an "old horse" and its recent impact?. In: Bertone J, editor. Equine geriatric medicine and surgery. St Louis (MO): WB Saunders; 2006. p. 1–4.
4. Harris PA. Review of equine feeding and stable management practices in the UK concentrating on the last decade of the 20th century. Equine Vet J Suppl 1999;28:46–54.
5. Chandler KJ, Mellor DJ. A pilot study of the prevalence of disease within a geriatric horse population. In: Proceedings of the 40th Congress of the British Equine Veterinary Association, Equine Vet J Ltd., Newmarket. 2001. p. 217.
6. Brosnahan MM, Paradis MR. Assessment of clinical characteristics, management practices, and activities of geriatric horses. J Am Vet Med Assoc 2003; 223:99–103.
7. McGowan TW. Aged horse health, management and welfare [PhD Thesis]. Queensland (Australia): University of Queensland; 2009.

8. Ireland JL, Clegg PD, McGowan CM, et al. A cross-sectional study of geriatric horses in the United Kingdom. Part 1: demographics and management practices. Equine Vet J 2011;43:30–6.
9. Hotchkiss JW, Reid SWJ, Christley RM. A survey of horse owners in Great Britain regarding horses in their care. Part 1: horse demographic characteristics and management. Equine Vet J 2007;39:294–300.
10. Wylie CE, Ireland JL, Collins SN, et al. Demographics and management practices of horses and ponies in Great Britain: a cross-sectional study. Res Vet Sci 2013;95:410–7.
11. Anon. U.S. Pet ownership & demographics sourcebook, 2007 edition. Schaumburg (IL): American Veterinary Medical Association; 2007.
12. Fortney WD. Geriatrics and aging. In: Hoskins J, editor. Geriatrics and gerontology of the dog and cat. 2nd edition. St Louis (MO): Saunders; 2004. p. 1–4.
13. Timiras PS. Old age as a stage of life: Common terms related to aging and methods used to study aging. In: Physiological basis of aging and geriatrics. 4th edition. New York: Informa Healthcare; 2007. p. 3–10.
14. Kinsella K, Phillips DR. Global aging: the challenge of success. Popul Bull 2005; 60:3–45.
15. Mellor DJ, Love S, Gettinby G, et al. Demographic characteristics of the equine population of northern Britain. Vet Rec 1999;145:299–304.
16. Hotchkiss JW. Quantitative epidemiological studies on recurrent airway obstruction in the horse population of Great Britain using a risk-screening questionnaire [PhD Thesis]. Glasgow (United Kingdom): University of Glasgow; 2004.
17. McGowan TW, Pinchbeck GL, Phillips C, et al. A survey of aged horses in Queensland, Australia. Part 1: management and preventive health care. Aust Vet J 2010;88:420–7.
18. Cole FL, Hodgson DR, Reid SWJ, et al. Owner-reported equine health disorders: results of an Australia-wide postal survey. Aust Vet J 2005;83:490–5.
19. Bushell R, Murray J. A survey of senior equine management: Owner practices and confidence. Livest Sci 2016;186:69–77.
20. Mellor DJ, Reid SWJ, Love S, et al. Sentinel practice-based survey of the management and health of horses in northern Britain. Vet Rec 2001;149:417–23.
21. Tomassini C. Demographic profile. Focus on Older People: office For national statistics: chapter 1. 2005. Available at: http://www.google.co.uk/url? sa=t&rct=j&q=&esrc=s&source=web&cd=1&cad=rja&uact=8&ved=0ahUK Ewjdkarzjs_MAhUGJsAKHeV5CLcQFggcMAA&url=http%3A%2F%2Fweb.ons. gov.uk%2Fons%2Frel%2Fmortality-ageing%2Ffocus-on-older-people%2F2005-edition%2Ffocus-on-older-people.pdf&usg=AFQjCNFiK-g-nRokuf_3xQv6oCdK Zo0gyA&bvm=bv.121421273,d.ZGg. Accessed May 10, 2016.
22. Anon. USDA/APHIS part 1: baseline reference of equine health and management. Fort Collins (CO): National Animal Health Monitoring System; 2005. p. 1–60.
23. Ireland JL, McGowan CM, Clegg PD, et al. A survey of health care and disease in geriatric horses aged 30 years or older. Vet J 2011;192:57–64.
24. Williams N. Disease conditions in geriatric horses. Equine Pract 2000;22:32.
25. Silva AG, Furr MO. Diagnoses, clinical pathology findings, and treatment outcome of geriatric horses: 345 cases (2006–2010). J Am Vet Med Assoc 2013;243:1762–8.
26. Kaneene JB, Saffell M, Fedewa DJ, et al. The Michigan equine monitoring system. 1. Design, implementation and population estimates. Prev Vet Med 1997; 29:263–75.

27. Codron E, Benamou-Smith A. Panorama of equine geriatrics. In: Proceedings of the 9th Congress of the World Equine Veterinary Association. Marrakech; 2006. p. 391–2.
28. Ralston SL, Squires EL, Nockels CF. Digestion in the aged horse. J Equine Vet Sci 1989;9:203–5.
29. Ralston SL, Breuer LH. Field evaluation of a feed formulated for geriatric horses. J Equine Vet Sci 1996;16:334–8.
30. Ralston SL, Christensen RA, Malinowski K, et al. Chronic effects of equine growth hormone (eGH) on intake, digestibility and retention of nutrients in aged mares. J Anim Sci 1996;74(Suppl 1):194.
31. Ralston SL, Malinowski K, Christensen RA, et al. Digestion in aged horses - Revisited. J Equine Vet Sci 2001;21:310–1.
32. Elzinga S, Nielsen BD, Schott HC, et al. Comparison of nutrient digestibility between adult and aged horses. J Equine Vet Sci 2014;34:1164–9.
33. McGowan TW, Pinchbeck GL, Phillips C, et al. A survey of aged horses in Queensland, Australia. Part 2: clinical signs and owner perceptions of health and welfare. Aust Vet J 2010;88:465–71.
34. Ireland JL, Clegg PD, McGowan CM, et al. A cross-sectional study of geriatric horses in the United Kingdom. Part 2: health care and disease. Equine Vet J 2011;43:37–44.
35. Ireland JL, Clegg PD, McGowan CM, et al. Disease prevalence in geriatric horses in the United Kingdom: veterinary clinical assessment of 200 cases. Equine Vet J 2012;44:101–6.
36. Adams AA, Sturgill TL, Breathnach CC, et al. Humoral and cell-mediated immune responses of old horses following recombinant canarypox virus vaccination and subsequent challenge infection. Vet Immunol Immunopathol 2011;139:128–40.
37. Ireland JL, Wylie CE, Collins SN, et al. Preventive health care and owner-reported disease prevalence of horses and ponies in Great Britain. Res Vet Sci 2013;95:418–24.
38. Koskinen HI. A survey of horse owner's compliance with the Finnish vaccination program. J Equine Vet Sci 2014;34:1114–7.
39. Ireland JL. Equine geriatric health and welfare in the United Kingdom [PhD Thesis]. Liverpool (United Kingdom): University of Liverpool; 2011.
40. Proudman CJ, Holmes MA, Sheoran AS, et al. Immunoepidemiology of the equine tapeworm Anoplocephala perfoliata: age-intensity profile and age-dependency of antibody subtype responses. Parasitology 1997;114:89–94.
41. McFarlane D, Hale GM, Johnson EM, et al. Fecal egg counts after anthelmintic administration to aged horses and horses with pituitary pars intermedia dysfunction. J Am Vet Med Assoc 2010;236:330–4.
42. Adams AA, Betancourt A, Barker VD, et al. Comparison of the immunologic response to anthelmintic treatment in old versus middle-aged horses. J Equine Vet Sci 2015;35:873–81.e3.
43. Shettko DL. The equine geriatric foot. In: Bertone J, editor. Equine geriatric medicine and surgery. St Louis (MO): WB Saunders; 2006. p. 217–21.
44. Anon. Equine industry welfare guidelines compendium for horses, ponies and donkey. 2nd edition. Banbury (United Kingdom): National Equine Welfare Council; 2005.
45. Perlman RM. The aging syndrome. J Am Geriatr Soc 1951;2:123–9.
46. Paradis MR. Demographics of health and disease in the geriatric horse. Vet Clin North Am Equine Pract 2002;18:391–401.

47. Hintz HF. The geriatric horse. Equine Pract 1995;17:8–10.
48. Lee M. Global health and population aging. Today's research on aging 4. Population Reference Bureau; 2007. Available at: www.prb.org/pdf07/todaysresearchaging4.pdf. Accessed May 10, 2016.
49. Fries JF. Aging, natural death and the compression of morbidity. N Engl J Med 1980;303:130–5.
50. Loeser RF. Age-related changes in the musculoskeletal system and the development of osteoarthritis. Clin Geriatr Med 2010;26:371–86.
51. Baker JR, Ellis CE. A survey of post-mortem findings in 480 horses 1958 to 1980: (1) Causes of death. Equine Vet J 1981;13:43–6.
52. Egenvall A, Penell JC, Bonnett BN, et al. Mortality of Swedish horses with complete life insurance between 1997 and 2000: variations with sex, age, breed and diagnosis. Vet Rec 2006;158:397–406.
53. Wallin L, Strandberg E, Philipsson J, et al. Estimates of longevity and causes of culling and death in Swedish warmblood and coldblood horses. Livest Prod Sci 2000;63:275–89.
54. Stevens KB, Marr CM, Horn JNR, et al. Effect of left-sided valvular regurgitation on mortality and causes of death among a population of middle-aged and older horses. Vet Rec 2009;164:6–10.
55. Ireland JL, Clegg PD, McGowan CM, et al. Factors associated with mortality of geriatric horses in the United Kingdom. Prev Vet Med 2011;101:204–18.
56. Leblond A, Villard I, Leblond L, et al. A retrospective evaluation of the causes of death of 448 insured French horses in 1995. Vet Res Commun 2000;24:85–102.
57. Kaneene JB, Ross WA, Miller R. The Michigan equine monitoring system. II. Frequencies and impact of selected health problems. Prev Vet Med 1997;29:277–92.
58. Buckley P, Dunn T, More SJ. Owners' perceptions of the health and performance of Pony Club horses in Australia. Prev Vet Med 2004;63:121–33.
59. Keegan KG, Dent EV, Wilson DA, et al. Repeatability of subjective evaluation of lameness in horses. Equine Vet J 2010;42:92–7.
60. Alford P, Geller S, Richardson B, et al. A multicenter, matched case-control study of risk factors for equine laminitis. Prev Vet Med 2001;49:209–22.
61. Slater MR, Hood DM, Carter GK. Descriptive epidemiological study of equine laminitis. Equine Vet J 1995;27:364–7.
62. Polzer J, Slater MR. Age, breed, sex and seasonality as risk factors for equine laminitis. Prev Vet Med 1997;29:179–84.
63. van der Kolk JH, Kalsbveek HC, van Garderen E, et al. Equine pituitary neoplasia: a clinical report of 21 cases (1990–1992). Vet Rec 1993;133:594–7.
64. Hillyer MH, Taylor FGR, Mair TS, et al. Diagnosis of hyperadrenocorticism in the horse. Equine Vet Educ 1992;4:131–4.
65. Donaldson MT, Jorgensen AJ, Beech J. Evaluation of suspected pituitary pars intermedia dysfunction in horses with laminitis. J Am Vet Med Assoc 2004;224:1123–7.
66. Karikoski NP, Horn I, McGowan TW, et al. The prevalence of endocrinopathic laminitis among horses presented for laminitis at a first-opinion/referral equine hospital. Domest Anim Endocrinol 2011;41:111–7.
67. Vemming DC, Steenkamp G, Carstens A, et al. Prevalence of dental disorders in an abattoir population of horses in South Africa by oral examination of intact and bisected heads. Vet J 2015;205:110–2.

68. Southwood LL, Gassert T, Lindborg S. Colic in geriatric compared to mature non-geriatric horses. Part 2: Treatment, diagnosis and short-term survival. Equine Vet J 2010;42:628–35.
69. Campbell ML, Colahan PC, Brown MP, et al. Cecal impaction in the horse. J Am Vet Med Assoc 1984;184:950–9.
70. Dart AJ, Hodgson DR, Snyder JR. Caecal disease in equids. Aust Vet J 1997;75: 552–7.
71. White JLN. Risk factors associated with colic. In: Robinson N, editor. Current therapy in equine medicine. 4th edition. St Louis (MO): WB Saunders; 1997. p. 174–9.
72. Hillyer MH, Taylor FGR, Proudman CJ, et al. Case control study to identify risk factors for simple colonic obstruction and distension colic in horses. Equine Vet J 2002;34:455–63.
73. Blikslager AT, Bowman KF, Haven ML, et al. Pedunculated lipomas as a cause of intestinal obstruction in horses: 17 cases (1983-1990). J Am Vet Med Assoc 1992;223:99–103.
74. Edwards GB, Proudman CJ. An analysis of 75 cases of intestinal obstruction caused by pedunculated lipomas. Equine Vet J 1994;26:18–21.
75. Freeman DE, Schaeffer DJ. Age distributions of horses with strangulation of the small intestine by a lipoma or in the epiploic foramen: 46 cases (1994-2000). J Am Vet Med Assoc 2001;219:87–9.
76. Garcia-Seco E, Wilson DA, Kramer J, et al. Prevalence and risk factors associated with outcome of surgical removal of pedunculated lipomas in horses: 102 cases (1987-2002). J Am Vet Med Assoc 2005;226:1529–37.
77. Krista KM, Kuebelbeck KL. Comparison of survival rates for geriatric horses versus nongeriatric horses following exploratory celiotomy for colic. J Am Vet Med Assoc 2009;235:1069–72.
78. Proudman CJ, Smith JE, Edwards GB, et al. Long-term survival of equine surgical colic cases. Part 2: modelling post-operative survival. Equine Vet J 2002;34: 438–43.
79. Proudman CJ, Edwards GB, Barnes J, et al. Factors affecting long-term survival of horses recovering from surgery of the small intestine. Equine Vet J 2005;37: 360–5.
80. Proudman CJ, Edwards GB, Barnes J, et al. Modelling long- term survival of horses following surgery for large intestinal disease. Equine Vet J 2005;37: 366–70.
81. Wheeler RG, Christley RM, McGowan CM. Prevalence of owner- reported respiratory disease in Pony Club horses. Vet Rec 2002;150:79–81.
82. Hotchkiss JW, Reid SWJ, Christley RM. A survey of horse owners in Great Britain regarding horses in their care. Part 2: Risk factors for recurrent airway obstruction. Equine Vet J 2007;39:301–8.
83. Ireland JL, Christley RM, McGowan CM, et al. Prevalence of and risk factors for recurrent airway obstruction in geriatric horses and ponies. Equine Vet J Suppl 2015;48:25.
84. Rettmer H, Hoffman AM, Lanz S, et al. Owner-reported coughing and nasal discharge are associated with clinical findings, arterial oxygen tension, mucus score and bronchoprovocation in horses with recurrent airway obstruction in a field setting. Equine Vet J 2015;47:291–5.
85. Marr CM, Bowen M. Cardiac disease in the geriatric horse. In: Bertone J, editor. Equine geriatric medicine and surgery. St Louis (MO): WB Saunders; 2006. p. 39–49.

86. Davis JL, Gardner SY, Schwabenton B, et al. Congestive heart failure in horses: 14 cases (1984–2001). J Am Vet Med Assoc 2002;220:1512–5.

87. Else RW, Holmes JR. Cardiac pathology in the horse: 1. Gross pathology. Equine Vet J 1972;4:2.

88. McFarlane D, Dybdal N, Donaldson MT, et al. Nitration and increased alpha-synuclein expression associated with dopaminergic neurodegeneration in equine pituitary *pars intermedia* dysfunction. J Neuroendocrinol 2005;17:73–80.

89. McFarlane D. Advantages and limitations of the equine disease, pituitary pars intermedia dysfunction as a model of spontaneous dopaminergic neurodegenerative disease. Ageng Res Rev 2007;6:54–63.

90. McCue PM. Equine Cushing's disease. Vet Clin North Am Equine Pract 2002;18: 533–43.

91. Schott HC. Pituitary pars intermedia dysfunction: equine Cushing's disease. Vet Clin North Am Equine Pract 2002;18:237–70.

92. McFarlane D. Equine pituitary pars intermedia dysfunction. Vet Clin North Am Equine Pract 2011;27:93–113.

93. McGowan TW, Pinchbeck GP, McGowan CM. Prevalence, risk factors and clinical signs predictive for equine pituitary pars intermedia dysfunction in aged horses. Equine Vet J 2013;45:74–9.

94. Frank N, Andrews FM, Sommardahl CS, et al. Evaluation of the combined dexamethasone suppression/thyrotropin-releasing hormone stimulation test for detection of pars intermedia pituitary adenomas in horses. J Vet Intern Med 2006;20:987–93.

95. Chandler KJ, Billson FM, Mellor DJ. Ophthalmic lesions in 83 geriatric horses and ponies. Vet Rec 2003;153:319–22.

96. Ireland JL, Clegg PD, McGowan CM, et al. Comparison of owner-reported health problems with veterinary assessment of geriatric horses in the United Kingdom. Equine Vet J 2012;44:94–100.

97. Cotchin E. A general survey of tumours in the horse. Equine Vet J 1977;9:16–21.

98. Yoshikawa H, Oishi H, Sumi A, et al. Spontaneous pituitary adenomas of the pars intermedia in 5 aged horses: Histopathological, immunohistochemical and ultrastructural studies. J Equine Sci 2001;12:119–26.

99. Junge RE, Sundberg JP, Lancaster WD. Papillomas and squamous cell carcinomas of horses. J Am Vet Med Assoc 1984;185:656–9.

100. Ueki H, Kowatari Y, Oyamada T, et al. Non- functional C-cell adenoma in aged horses. J Comp Pathol 2004;131:157–65.

101. Meyer J, DeLay J, Bienzle D. Clinical, laboratory and histopathologic features of equine lymphoma. Vet Pathol 2006;43:914–24.

102. Sweeney CR, Gillette DM. Thoracic neoplasia in equids: 35 cases (1967-1987). J Am Vet Med Assoc 1989;195:374–7.

103. Mair TS, Brown PJ. Clinical and pathologic features of thoracic neoplasia in the horse. Equine Vet J 1993;25:220–3.

Dental Disease in Aged Horses and Its Management

Victoria M. Nicholls, BVetMed, Cert AVP (EM), Cert AVP (ED), MRCVS[a],
Neil Townsend, MSc, BVSc, Cert ES (Soft Tissue), MRCVS[b],*

KEYWORDS

- Dental disease • Geriatric dentistry • Equine

KEY POINTS

- Dental disorders are common in the equine geriatric population.
- Age-related changes in normal equine dentition result in dental disorders.
- Geriatric patients have specific requirements for restraint and sedation.
- A key point is ensuring oral comfort and maximizing masticatory ability.
- Dental treatment in geriatric patients often requires concurrent management changes, such a dietary modification and treatment of coexisting problems, such as pituitary pars intermedia dysfunction (PPID).

INTRODUCTION

There have been many recent articles focused on geriatric equine veterinary care, which have enhanced knowledge of age-related dental disease and how to tailor specific care toward this significant and potentially increasing proportion of the equine population.[1–5] From recent studies, it is known that horses[5] and donkeys[6] have an increased prevalence of dental disorders, in particular periodontal disease, from 15 years of age. Furthermore, donkeys older than 20 years of age are known to have an increased prevalence of wear abnormalities, cheek tooth displacements and diastemata, and loss of teeth (**Fig. 1**), along with other dental abnormalities, such as shear mouth and smooth mouth.[7] Because dental abnormalities have been documented as present in 95.4% of geriatric animals,[4] there is absolute justification for early intervention and preventive care in the equid population, in addition to the unequivocal requirement for routine dental care for the older geriatric proportion. So why is the geriatric population over-represented in terms of dental disorders?

[a] Veterinary Postgraduate Unit, University of Liverpool, School of Veterinary Science, Leahurst, Neston CH64 7TE, UK; [b] Three Counties Equine Hospital, Stratford Bridge, Ripple, Tewksbury, Gloucestershire GL20 6HE, UK
* Corresponding author.
E-mail address: neil.townsend@tceh.co.uk

Vet Clin Equine 32 (2016) 215–227
http://dx.doi.org/10.1016/j.cveq.2016.04.002
0749-0739/16/$ – see front matter © 2016 Elsevier Inc. All rights reserved.

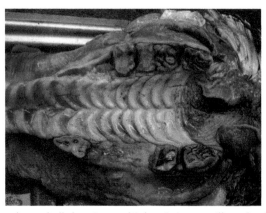

Fig. 1. A geriatric cadaver skull showing multiple missing maxillary cheek teeth.

ANATOMIC CHANGES WITH AGING

Normal age-related changes in equine dentition are a major contributing factor to geriatric dental disorders due to their hypsodont nature, which translates into a finite length of tooth for eruption. Various factors, such as dietary management and excessive dental treatment, may also decrease the functional length of the tooth and exacerbate normal age-related changes.[8]

Equid teeth have a normal taper from the occlusal surface to the apex, and the cheek teeth are tightly packed together as a single grinding unit by the opposing angulation of the 06s, 10s, and 11s. As the horse ages and the teeth erupt, they become smaller on cross-section, with the incisors beginning as oval-shaped after eruption, becoming triangular thereafter, and finally becoming oval-shaped as the horse matures. Eventually the tapering predisposes the horse to development of senile diastemata between both the incisors and the cheek teeth, with secondary food impaction and periodontal disease.[9]

All teeth have the presence of enamel, dentine, and cementum on their occlusal surface, and exposure of all 3 is essential for efficient mastication. The differential wear in these structures allows the formation of enamel ridges and acts as a self-sharpening mechanism. The maxillary cheek teeth have 2 separate infundibulae (enamel cups) (**Fig. 2**) in the center of the tooth, and the mandibular cheek teeth have pronounced infolding of the peripheral enamel to increase the grinding area of the tooth. As the tooth matures, the infundibulae wear out and the enamel infolding becomes less prominent, leading to only a thin shell of peripheral enamel left around the tooth (cupped-out tooth) (see **Fig. 2**). Eventually the peripheral enamel wears away at the junction of the individual roots, leaving a smooth occlusal surface (smooth mouth), which is inefficient at mastication, has no wear resistance, and may be quickly worn away.

In a further exacerbation of problems for geriatric patients, there is also an age-related change in occlusal contact. Biomechanical studies have demonstrated that the equine mandibular cheek teeth become more curved rostrocaudally but did not change their dental position in the mouth with aging. This is in contrast to the maxillary cheek teeth, which changed only their mesio-occlusal angle (ie, their dental position) but did not become more curved rostrocaudally. This effectively means that the occlusal contact between the cheek teeth changes with aging and may contribute to the wear pattern disorders commonly seen in geriatric dental patients, such as wave mouth and senile diastemata.

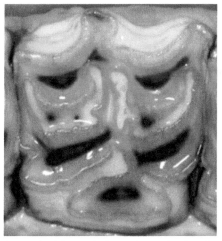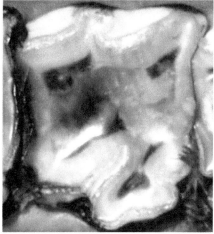

Fig. 2. The left tooth shows the occlusal surface of a normal maxillary cheek tooth. The right tooth shows the occlusal surface of maxillary cheek tooth, which has worn away its infundibular enamel, leaving only the peripheral enamel.

EXAMINATION OF THE GERIATRIC PATIENT

Geriatric patients require a full medical history and thorough clinical examination to rule out concurrent disease; these may represent the only opportunity to perform a geriatric health check in these animals and ascertain the presence of underlying systemic disease, such as PPID (**Fig. 3**) or cardiac disease. It is particularly important to evaluate the horse for subtle indicators of dental disease, such as epiphora, nasal discharge, muscle asymmetry, and specifically chronic nonhealing mucosal ulceration, which may be indicative of PPID, which is more common in the geriatric patient.[4,5]

Cardiac disease and orthopedic problems, such as arthritis and muscle weakness, need to be considered when sedating and restraining geriatric animals for dental examination. These animals tend to have increased sensitivity and decreased clearance of the commonly used sedative agents[10] so a lower dose may be indicated. Also consider combining the sedative protocol with opioids to produce

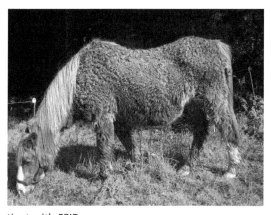

Fig. 3. Geriatric patient with PPID.

neuroleptanalgesia; the synergistic properties result in superior analgesia, potentially fewer side effects, and less ataxia[11] compared with a single-agent approach (**Box 1**).[12]

Currently, the authors use low dosages of α_2-adrenoreceptor agonists (either detomidine or romifidine) in combination with either butorphanol tartrate or morphine sulphate. Continuous rate infusion of either xylazine or detomidine also may be used. Where possible, these animals should be placed in stocks or backed into a corner because they tend to slump down on their forelimbs, particularly when their head is supported on a stand or sling (**Fig. 4**).

Locoregional anesthesia can also be used as part of multimodal layered approach to analgesia[11] and can potentially reduce the total volume of sedation. Commonly used regional blocks for dentistry include maxillary, inferior alveolar, mental, and infraorbital nerve blocks. At the conclusion of the procedure or during unstimulated periods, the heavily sedated geriatric should be monitored closely, because it is the author's experience that they are more prone to profound ataxia.

It is also important to consider a patient's underlying immune status and ensure that adequate antibiotic and tetanus cover are considered, particularly in cases of suspected or confirmed PPID.

Clinical signs of dental disease vary with the severity of the pathology, although a significant proportion of equids show no clinical signs despite the presence of multiple dental abnormalities. In severe cases, quidding may be evident and the animals may take longer to masticate. Temporary cheek swellings may be present if forage becomes packed between the cheek and the teeth (**Fig. 5**) and long fibers may be present in the feces. Over a period of time, these animals may be noted to show weight loss associated with decreased food intake and inefficient digestion.

COMMON DENTAL DISORDERS OF AGED EQUIDS
Disorders of the Incisor Teeth

Age-related wear patterns of the incisors are common as the contact angle between the mandibular and maxillary incisors becomes more acute. This can affect normal prehension and the diet may require subsequent modification. Nonetheless, geriatric patients seem to function well despite a complete lack of incisor contact if their diet and calorific intake is managed appropriately.

As with younger horses, the incisors of geriatric animals are prone to excessive wear due to behavioral problems, such as cribbing and wind-sucking. If teeth are lost, malocclusions may develop, with overgrowth of the opposing tooth and often displacement of the remaining teeth, and regular reduction of the overgrown incisor is required to maintain normal occlusion. It is advisable to reduce overgrown incisors in stages, several months apart, to avoid pulpar exposure.

Box 1
Key restraint differences for geriatric patients

- Low-dose sedation: increased sensitivity and decreased clearance
- α_2-Agonist + butorphanol/morphine
- Stocks/backed into corner
- Use regional anesthesia if possible
- Premedication with analgesics *before* procedure where possible
- Tetanus prophylaxis
- Antibiotics, particularly if concurrent PPID

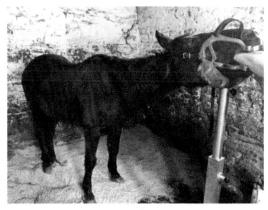

Fig. 4. Geriatric patient with head supported for cheek tooth extraction.

The occlusal surface of geriatric incisors is often abnormal, with the development of a ventral convex curvature (smile), a dorsal convex curvature (frown), or a diagonal surface (slope or slant mouth). These changes are form due to abnormal mastication, usually as a result of cheek teeth problems, although smile mouth may be regarded as a normal finding in aged donkeys.[6] Once the cheek teeth abnormalities have been corrected, the incisor curvature may be addressed.

The tapering of the incisor teeth toward the apical region may lead to the development of senile diastemata in several geriatric horses (**Fig. 6**). This may lead to food impaction and secondary periodontal disease, although because these teeth are not subjected to huge masticatory forces, they rarely develop deep periodontal pockets. The impacted food can be easily cleared by most owners using a standard toothbrush, although particularly narrow or valve diastemata may be widened with a rotating diastema burr.

A more important disorder in terms of effective mastication is the recently reported equine odontoclastic tooth resorption and hypercementosis (EOTRH) disorder. This is a more severe form of incisor periodontal disease recognized in geriatric patients and is associated with radiographically lytic changes and cemental hyperplasia.[13] The precise etiology is unknown but it primarily affects the intra-alveolar aspect of the teeth,

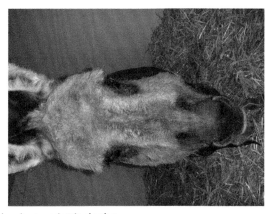

Fig. 5. Food packing in a geriatric donkey.

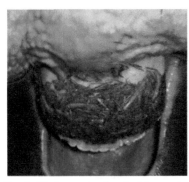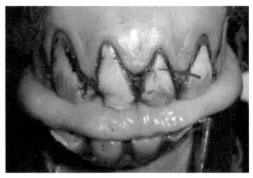

Fig. 6. Photograph of an incisive region showing food packing between teeth (*left*) and underlying senile diastemata once the food is removed (*right*).

with odontoclastic cells causing resorptive lesions extending into enamel, dentin, and cementum, causing loss of the normal tooth architecture.

Initially affected horses present with mild gingival inflammation and edema, although, with progression, draining tracts may develop in the gingiva and there may be gingival swelling and recession. These signs are usually accompanied by hypercementosis of the reserve crown and apex. Eventually the interdental bone becomes lytic and the incisors become loose. These horses may present with varying clinical signs with some presenting only with hypercementosis, whereas some present with pain on mastication, particularly if the teeth are loose (**Fig. 7**). The authors' experience of treating these cases with long-term antibiotics and anti-inflammatories has been unsuccessful and staged removal of loose incisors is now their treatment of choice.

Disorders of the Canine Teeth

Calculus accumulation and mild periodontal disease are the most common disorders of the canine teeth, and these are easily treated with forceps removal of the calculus accumulation. Extremely large accumulations of calculus around the mandibular incisors can be associated tongue ulcers. These teeth may also become fractured or damaged, necessitating removal using either elevation or surgical techniques.[14]

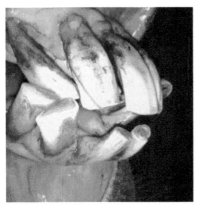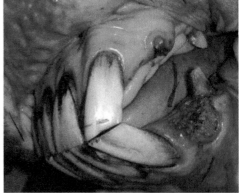

Fig. 7. Photographs illustrating spectrum of severity of EOTRH. The horse on the left was relatively asymptomatic compared with the horse on the right that presented with great difficulty eating.

Disorders of the Cheek Teeth

Geriatric horses suffer from the same abnormalities of wear as younger horses, although usually at a more advanced stage, with step mouth, wave mouth, and shear mouth all present. Overgrown teeth tend to be complicated by the lack of reserve crown to the tooth and may be unstable in the alveolus leading to displacement or loss of these teeth. Smooth mouth is seen in geriatric animals when the teeth become inefficient grinding units. A study looking at the prevalence of cheek tooth disorders in animals greater than or equal to 15 years old has shown the most prevalent dental pathologies to be mandibular lingual enamel points (64%), maxillary buccal enamel points (51%), periodontal disease (42.9%), and cheek teeth diastemata (41.9%), with the prevalence of wave mouth (**Fig. 8**), step mouth, smooth mouth (**Fig. 9**), diastemata (**Fig. 10**), and periodontal disease all significantly increased with increasing age.[4] A similar study looking at very old animals, greater than or equal to 30 years old, has shown similarly high prevalence of dental disorders, with cheek teeth diastemata (78.7%), periodontal disease (75%), and smooth mouth (71.7%) the most prevalent.[5] Similar prevalence of dental disease has been shown in geriatric donkeys.[6]

Treatment of cheek teeth disorders in geriatric animals is often limited due to the lack of reserve crown. As much of the occlusal crown should be preserved to allow efficient mastication, although all sharp points that may contact the oral soft tissues should be removed (usually the buccal aspect of the maxillary cheek teeth and the lingual aspect of the mandibular cheek teeth). Excessively large teeth should be reduced in stages to prevent pulpar exposure and with great care because these teeth may be unstable within the alveolus. Overgrown, slightly loose teeth may firmly reattach once the overgrowth is removed. Severely displaced teeth should be extracted if associated with soft tissue trauma or marked periodontal disease. Digitally loose teeth should be extracted orally where possible.

Extraoral Pathology

Temporomandibular joint (TMJ) pathology, although common in humans,[15] is uncommonly diagnosed in equine patients.[16] This may not be due to a low prevalence of disease but because definitely diagnosing TMJ pathology in horses potentially is difficult. Clinical signs associated with TMJ osteoarthritis include a decreased range of mandibular motion and a preference to chew on the nonaffected side (with the subsequent development of a shear mouth on the affected side). Joint distension and bony

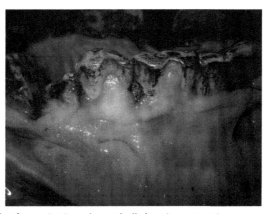

Fig. 8. Photograph of a geriatric cadaver skull showing extensive wave mouth formation.

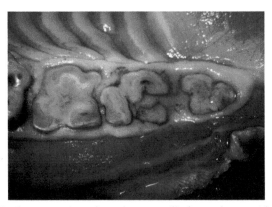

Fig. 9. Photograph of a proportion of a cadaver maxilla from a horse with a smooth mouth. Note how the 07 has been worn away to its constituent roots.

swelling over the affected joint may also be present, with masseter muscle atrophy present in chronic cases.

A definitive diagnosis can be reached with intrasynovial anesthesia of the affected TMJ using previously described approaches.[17,18] Imaging of the equine TMJ is difficult although radiographic projections,[19,20] ultrasonographic examination,[21,22] scintigraphic examination,[18] and CT examination[23] have been described. Treatment options for TMJ arthropathy include intra-articular medication with corticosteroids, arthroscopic exploration,[24] and mandibular condylectomy and meniscectomy.[25] Difficulty in mastication may also be due to osteoarthritis of the temporohyoid joint, which has recently been shown to develop age-related pathology.[26]

The frequency of occurrence of equine oral and sinonasal neoplasia remains low because they are often difficult to diagnose at an early stage, which makes subsequent treatment often complicated.[27–30] Specifically, the incidence of neoplasia in geriatric equine populations is difficult to ascertain by a generalized lack of routine examination and poor recognition of often nonspecific signs, such as ocular and nasal discharge, dysmastication, respiratory signs, and weight loss. Furthermore, there may also be a reluctance to thoroughly investigate and subsequently attempt to treat these

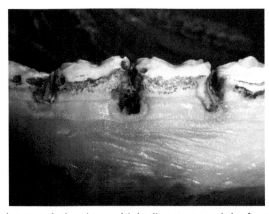

Fig. 10. Cadaver photograph showing multiple diastemata and the formation of extensive periodontal pockets.

geriatric patients due to financial constraints. What is clear from recent literature reports is that improved client education and preventive care of geriatric horses may lead to earlier detection of neoplasia and a more optimistic outlook for these patients.[31–33]

Management

The key aim of geriatric dental care is to ensure oral comfort and to maximize masticatory ability where possible. The short reserve crown limits in geriatric patients limit dental crown reduction and some of the disorders of wear may be longstanding. The mainstay of treatment must, therefore, revolve on preserving the masticatory ability by maintaining occlusal contact where possible rather than the perhaps more important alterations of the occlusal profile in younger patients.

Loose and missing teeth are far more common in the geriatric population than in younger horses due to the reduction in tooth stability as the reserve crown is reduced. Periodontal disease, often secondary to age-related senile diastemata, can contribute to loose or missing teeth due to associated periodontal ligament damage (**Fig. 11**). Although it is often tempting to extract loose cheek where present, it must be remembered that preservation of masticatory surfaces is always preferable where possible, and widespread extractions can effectively shorten a horse's life if not performed selectively. Extraction methods are beyond the scope of this review but it is important to reiterate the importance of using a multimodal approach to neuroleptanalgesia, regional anesthesia, and preemptive analgesia and tetanus prophylaxis.

The decrease in enamel thickness and enamel infolding further apically in teeth means less enamel is exposed on the occlusal surface as the teeth wear down, resulting in teeth that are not able to resist wear as effectively.[8] Teeth with only cementum and dentine remaining are ineffective at masticating fibrous food.[9] Furthermore, as the teeth wear and become narrower apically,[34] the occlusal surface area decreases, which, in combination with decreasing tooth angulation and compression forces, results in a failure to maintain close interdental contact. The result is subsequent senile diastemata formation.[9]

Diastemata and periodontal disease often involve the caudal cheek teeth and a dental mirror and light source are essential for complete evaluation. In geriatric animals, many diastema may be due to the anatomic tapering of the tooth toward

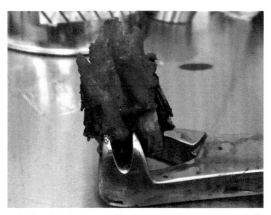

Fig. 11. A cheek tooth that has been orally extracted from a geriatric horse suffering from severe periodontal disease. Food can still be noted on the rostral and caudal margins of this tooth due to diastemata.

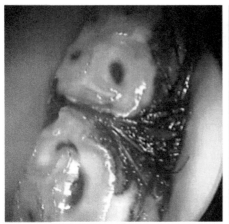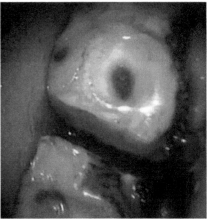

Fig. 12. The left image shows a valve type diastema between 310/311 with marked food pocketing. The right image shows the same diastema after flushing and diastema widening.

its apex and the loss of angulation of the rostral and caudal cheek teeth, so the cause cannot be eliminated. All periodontal pockets should be flushed clear of food material and the type of diastema and the severity of the periodontal disease assessed. If the diastema is narrower at the occlusal aspect than the gingival aspect, widening with a rotating diastema burr may improve the severity of the periodontal disease[35] (**Fig. 12**). Any exaggerated transverse ridges opposite the diastema should be reduced to decrease impaction of food into the diastemata.[36] Some investigators have advocated packing of the periodontal pockets with dental impression compound with or without antibiotic gel[37,38] but this has not been substantiated in clinical studies (**Fig. 13**).

Horses with smooth mouth are difficult to treat because any remaining enamel should be preserved as much as possible. All enamel points that may cause soft tissue damage should be reduced and the body condition score and the diet of the animal monitored closely (**Box 2**).

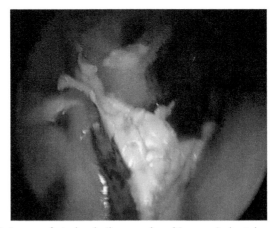

Fig. 13. Oroscopic image of vinyl polysiloxane placed in a periodontal pocket between 309 and 310.

Box 2
Considerations for management of geriatric dental patients

- Older horses have decreased masticatory force as a result of decrease in curve of Spee,[39] which, combined with smooth mouth and reduced enamel ridges, further reduces masticatory ability.

- Teeth with only cementum and dentine remaining are ineffective at masticating fibrous food.[9]

- Ensure fiber content sufficient for gastrointestinal health in addition to maintaining minimum daily energy intake.[8]

- High-quality roughage supplemented with minerals and vitamins (eg, balancer).[40]

- Fresh (young) grass is best fed to affected animals due high moisture content and lower levels acid fiber so minimal mastication and efficient digestion. Soaked fiber cubes can be fed in winter if grass is not available.

- Avoid short chop fiber if diastemata present.[8]

- Process cereal grains (eg, pelleting and extruding) to improve starch digestibility in the small intestine and avoid starch overload in the hindgut.[40]

- Consider testing early for PPID.

- Promote ease of consumption – reduce competition from other horses and address orthopedic issues that may impair movement, especially if grazing marginal pastures.

- Add oil to increase calorific intake.

- Monitor body condition score carefully and adjust rations accordingly.

Affected animals tend to do well in the summer months when grass is freely available but struggle in winter when asked to eat hay. The hay may be chopped (chaffed) or hay or grass cubes may be fed in 2 to 3 feeds per day. Complete and pelleted feeds are available, although they are expensive and require soaking to prevent choke. Vegetable oil may also be added to increase the calorific content. For a more detailed description of geriatric nutrition (McGregor Argo C: Nutritional Management of the Older Horse, in this issue).

SUMMARY

The recent awareness of geriatric equine conditions, as exemplified in the series of articles from this issue devoted to geriatric medicine, in conjunction with increased evidence-based, medicine-based diagnostics; adjunctive therapy; and surgery, is an encouraging prospect for geriatric veterinary care in the horse. The mainstay of geriatric dental care is to focus on early client education and preventive care with subsequent regular dental examinations and dietary management to ensure oral comfort and masticatory efficiency.

REFERENCES

1. Brosnahan MM, Paradis MR. Demographic and clinical characteristics of geriatric horses: 467 cases (1989 – 1999). J Am Vet Med Assoc 2003;223:93–103.

2. McGowan TW, Pinchbeck G, Phillips CJ, et al. A survey of aged horses in Queensland, Australia. Part 1: management and preventative health care. Aust Vet J 2010;88:420–7.

3. McGowan TW, Pinchbeck G, Phillips CJ, et al. A survey of aged horses in Queensland, Australia. Part 2: clinical signs and owners' perceptions of heath and welfare. Aust Vet J 2010;88:465–71.
4. Ireland JL, Clegg PD, McGowan CM, et al. Disease prevalence in geriatric horses in the United Kingdom: veterinary clinical assessment of 200 cases. Equine Vet J 2012;44:101–6.
5. Ireland JL, McGowan CM, Clegg PD, et al. A survey of health care and disease in geriatric horses aged 30 years or older. Vet J 2012;192:57–64.
6. Du Toit N, Burden FA, Dixon PM. Clinical dental examinations of 357 donkeys in the UK: part 1-prevalence of dental disorders. Equine Vet J 2009;41:390–4.
7. Du Toit N, Gallagher J, Burden FA, et al. Post mortem survey of dental disorders in 349 donkeys from an aged population (2005-2006). Part 1: prevalence of specific dental disorders. Equine Vet J 2008;40(3):204–8.
8. Du Toit N, Rucker BA. The gold standard of dental care: the geriatric horse. Vet Clin North Am Equine Pract 2013;29(2):5210527.
9. Dixon PM, Dacre I. A review of equine dental disorders. Vet J 2005;169(2): 165–87.
10. Donaldson LL. Anaesthetic considerations for the geriatric equine. In: Bertone J, editor. Equine geriatric medicine and surgery. St Louis (MO): Elsevier; 2006. p. 25–37.
11. Vigani A, Garcia-Pereira FL. Anaesthesia and analgesia for standing equine surgery. Vet Clin North Am Equine Pract 2014;30(1):1–17.
12. Dutton DW, Lashnits KJ, Wegner K. Managing severe hoof pain in a horse using multimodal analgesia and a modified composite pain score. Equine Vet Educ 2009;21(1):37–43.
13. Stasyk C, Biernert A, Kreutzer R, et al. Equine odontoclastic tooth resorption and hypercementosis. Vet J 2008;178:372–9.
14. Rawlinson JT, Earley E. Advances in the treatment of disease equine incisor and canine teeth. Vet Clin North Am Equine Pract 2013;29:411–40.
15. Rugh JD, Solberg WK. Oral health status in the United States: temporomandibular joint disorders. J Dent Educ 1985;49:398–405.
16. Ramzan PT. The temporomandibular joint: component of clinical complexity. Equine Vet J 2006;38(2):102–4.
17. Rosenstein DS, Bullock MF, Ocello PJ, et al. Arthrocentesis of the temporomandibular joint in adult horses. Am J Vet Res 2001;62:729–33.
18. Weller R, Cauvin ER, Bowen IM, et al. Comparison of radiography, scintigraphy and ultrasonography in the diagnosis of a case of temporomandibular joint arthropathy in a horse. Vet Rec 1999;144:377–9.
19. Ramzan PH, Marr CM, Meehan J, et al. Novel oblique radiographic projection of the temporomandibular articulation of horses. Vet Rec 2008;162:714–6.
20. Townsend NB, Cotton JC, Barakzai SZ. A tangential radiographic projection for investigation of the equine temporomandibular joint. Vet Surg 2009;38:601–6.
21. Weller R, Taylor S, Maierl J, et al. Ultrasonographic anatomy of the equine temporomandibular joint. Equine Vet J 1999;31:529–32.
22. Rodriguez MJ, Soler M, Lattore R, et al. Ultrasonographic anatomy of the temporomandibular joint in healthy pure-bred Spanish horses. Vet Radiol Ultrasound 2007;48:149–54.
23. Rodriguez MJ, Lattore R, Lopez-Albors O, et al. Computed tomographic anatomy of the temporomandibular joint in the young horse. Equine Vet J 2008;40:566–71.
24. Weller R, Maierl J, Bowen IM, et al. The arthroscopic approach and intra-articular anatomy of the equine temporomandibular joint. Equine Vet J 2002;34:421–4.

25. Nagy AD, Simhofer H. Mandibular condylectomy and meniscectomy for the treatment of septic temporomandibular joint arthritis in a horse. Vet Surg 2006;35: 663–8.
26. Naylor RJ, Perkins JD, Allen S, et al. Histopathology and computed tomography of age-associated degeneration of the equine temporohyoid joint. Equine Vet J 2010;42:425–30.
27. Dixon PM, Head KW. Equine nasal and paranasal sinus tumours: part 2: a contribution of 28 case reports. Vet J 1999;157:279–94.
28. Tremaine WH, Dixon PM. A long term study of 277 cases of equine sinonasal disease. Part 1: details of horses, historical, clinical and ancillary diagnostic findings. Equine Vet J 2001;33:274–82.
29. Tremaine WH, Dixon PM. A long term study of 277 cases of equine sinonasal disease. Part 2: treatments and results of treatments. Equine Vet J 2001;33:283–9.
30. Witte TH, Perkins JD. Early diagnosis may hold the key to the successful treatment of nasal and paranasal sinus neoplasia in the horse. Equine Vet Educ 2011;23:441–7.
31. Springer T, Elce YA, Green E. Treatment of an osteoblastic osteosarcoma in an aged gelding. Equine Vet Educ 2010;22:159–62.
32. Witte S, Mueller POE, Kosarek C, et al. Collision tumour affecting the paranasal sinuses of a geriatric donkey. Equine Vet Educ 2012;24:163–8.
33. Laus F, Rossi G, Paggi E, et al. Adenocarcinoma involving the tongue and the epiglottis in a horse. J Vet Med Sci 2014;76:467–70.
34. Dixon PM, Copeland AN. The radiological appearance of mandibular cheek teeth in ponies of different ages. Equine Vet Educ 1993;5:317–23.
35. Dixon PM, Barakzai S, Collins N, et al. Treatment of equine cheek teeth by mechanical widening of diastemata in 60 horses (2000-2006). Equine Vet J 2008;40:22–8.
36. Townsend NB, Barakzai S. Equine dentistry– dealing diastemata. UK vet 2008; 13:4–8.
37. Klugh DO. Equine periodontal disease. Clin Tech Equine Pract 2005;4:135–47.
38. Townsend NB. Is flushing and packing adequate for diastema treatment. Equine Vet Educ 2015;27:385–6.
39. Huthmann S, Gasse H, Jacob HG, et al. Biomechanical evaluation of equine masticatory action: position and curvature of equine cheek teeth and age-related changes. Anat Rec 2008;291(5):565–70.
40. Siciliano PD. Nutrition and feeding of the geriatric horse. Vet Clin North Am Equine Pract 2002;18(3):491–508.

Musculoskeletal Disease in Aged Horses and Its Management

Paul René van Weeren, DVM, PhD[a],*, Willem Back, DVM, PhD[a,b]

KEYWORDS

- Osteoarthritis • Laminitis • Geriatric horse • Pain management
- Degenerative joint disease

KEY POINTS

- Musculoskeletal disease is the most prevalent health and welfare issue in aged horses with osteoarthritis (OA) and chronic laminitis being the most common single disorders.
- The prevalence of OA is greater than 50% in horses older than 15 years and up to 80% to 90% in horses over 30.
- Management of OA in the elderly horse is multifocal and focuses, apart from pain management, also on optimizing the exercise regimen and improving living conditions.
- Laminitis in the geriatric horse is related to pituitary pars intermedia dysfunction (PPID) in many cases.
- Laminitis in geriatric horses is managed as in the general horse population, with additional benefit from pergolide administration in PPID cases.

INTRODUCTION

It is a well-known fact that musculoskeletal disease is the principal cause of wastage in the equine industry. More than 30 years ago, this was demonstrated in epidemiologic research in Thoroughbred racing.[1,2] More recently, Bertuglia and co-workers,[3] in a cohort of 356 Standardbreds, reported an overall exercise-related musculoskeletal injury rate of 4.79 per 100 horse-months, a figure substantially higher than the injury rate of 1.8 per 100 horse-months found in a prospective study in Thoroughbreds in training, although these injuries concerned joint-related injuries only.[4] Musculoskeletal disease-related wastage is not only in the racing breeds. In a study on 126 elite show jumpers, 55% and 22% of days lost to training for medical reasons were owing to non-acute and acute orthopedic injuries respectively.[5] Combined, this figure is similar to

The authors have nothing to disclose.
[a] Department of Equine Sciences, Faculty of Veterinary Medicine, Utrecht University, Yalelaan 112, 3584CM Utrecht, the Netherlands; [b] Department of Surgery and Anaesthesiology, Faculty of Veterinary Medicine, Ghent University, Salisburylaan 133, 9280 Merelbeke, Belgium
* Corresponding author.
E-mail address: R.VANWEEREN@UU.NL

the 72.1% of days lost in a study on racehorses in South Africa.[2] Even in young horses subjected to a standard riding horse quality test, moderate or severe orthopedic clinical findings were reported in 24% of cases, against only 6% moderate or severe clinical medical findings.[6] Of the musculoskeletal tissues (muscle, bone, joints, tendons/ligaments) the latter two are by far of greatest clinical relevance in most disciplines, mainly because of their poor healing capacity and the consequent tendency to develop chronic disorders.

In the aging human population, musculoskeletal disorders have a huge influence on quality of life and rank first as cause of years lived with disability.[7] Given the high prevalence of musculoskeletal disease in nongeriatric horses, as outlined, it is not surprising that this is the case for the elderly horse as well. In a study of 69 horses aged 30 years and older, a staggering 77% was found to be lame at clinical examination with virtually all (97%) having a reduced range of motion in at least 1 joint.[8] When reducing the age above which a horse was deemed to be geriatric to 15 years, these figures were still 51% and 84% in a population of 200 animals.[9] In this group, owners reported lameness only in 23% of cases (and reported hoof abnormalities in 27% against 80% diagnosed by the veterinarian).[10] Hence, owner perception of musculoskeletal problems in aging horses is significantly less than expert diagnosis, which is of great importance from both the veterinary and welfare perspectives. In line with these figures on the prevalence of musculoskeletal disease in the elderly horse, lameness was found to be the principal reason for euthanasia of geriatric horses (24%), just before colic (21%).[11]

The vast majority of lameness cases in geriatric horses are owing to chronic degenerative joint disease or osteoarthritis (OA), as evidenced by the high prevalence of reduced range of motion in 1 or more joints. This is similar to the human situation. Another frequent cause of disablement in the elderly horse that does not have a homologue in human medicine is (chronic) laminitis. Therefore, this review focuses on the clinical aspects and related care and management of chronic joint disorders (OA), and on how to deal with laminitis in the elderly horse. Because pain management is an important common aspect of both conditions, it is an area of focus in this review.

CHRONIC JOINT DISEASE OR OSTEOARTHRITIS IN THE GERIATRIC HORSE
Definition, Pathogenesis, and Clinical Signs

Equine OA has been defined as a group of disorders characterized by a common end stage, namely, progressive deterioration of the articular cartilage accompanied by changes in the bone and soft tissues of the joint.[12] The basic pathogenic mechanism of OA is a disturbance of the joint homeostasis leading to an imbalance of the anabolic and catabolic processes in the joint. Whereas damage to the articular cartilage is among the hallmarks of OA and is generally seen as emblematic for the disease, it is not the only tissue that is affected. In OA, the subchondral bone is also affected and changes in the subchondral bone have even been suggested to be primary events rather than secondary ones.[13] The synovial membrane is also involved and the composition of the synovial fluid will be altered to a certain extent, reflecting the current concept of seeing the joint as a complex multicomposite organ, rather than as a structure consisting of a variety of separately reacting tissue types.[14]

There are various etiologic factors involved in OA, including synovitis, single events producing major joint trauma, and repeated microtrauma as a result of repeated overloading. In the horse, the last 2 pathways are probably most important with use-related wear and tear being highly prevalent. In a post mortem study using

50 metacarpophalangeal joints from racehorses one-third of all 2- and 3-year-old horses had partial- or full-thickness cartilage lesions and signs of OA; the severity of OA increased until age 6.[15] Once OA has commenced, it tends to advance slowly but inexorably in severity and to spread over the joint. In the horse, this process has been investigated in the metacarpophalangeal joint by determining the so-called Cartilage Degeneration Index, a technique based on the fact that Indian ink particles will be retained by damaged, but not by intact, cartilage (**Fig. 1**).[16,17] Independent of the cause of OA, the end stage is common and it is often end stage disease that is encountered in geriatric horses (**Fig. 2**).

OA is an insidious disease par excellence. Articular cartilage is aneural and the damage may have become substantial before pain to some degree is perceived through triggering of nerve endings in the subchondral bone, the very richly innervated periosteum at the joint margins, or the synovial membrane. Nevertheless, articular homeostasis will already be disturbed before this stage as a sequel to the catabolic processes that are ongoing in the cartilage layer, which will result in low-grade inflammation that may become clinically apparent as joint effusion. A typical characteristic of the clinical features of OA is its intermittent character. Horses may be lameness free for a long period and then, mostly because of inadvertent overloading, suddenly become symptomatic with joint effusion and lameness. These signs tend to wear off over time, but, if no treatment is installed, this may take a long time. A more consistent clinical feature is the often a substantial decrease in joint range of motion, which is a very frequent finding in the older horse, as noted.[8] This is caused by stiffening of the periarticular structures and joint capsule and by the osteophytes that frequently form at the joint margins. These are structural changes that do not wear off with time, but tend to become more severe with advancing age. Whereas the diagnosis of OA in the geriatric horse will in general not present problems, because it often represents end-stage disease, the sustainable management of the condition is a greater challenge.

Pain in Osteoarthritis

Pain is the major symptom of OA in humans.[18] It has been described as "the most prominent, but least well-studied feature of OA."[19] Basic knowledge of the physiologic

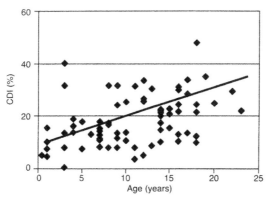

Fig. 1. Correlation between the cartilage degeneration index (CDI; %) of the proximal articular cartilage surface of the first phalanx and age of the horses (years; $r = 0.41$; $P<.001$). Regression line indicated. (*From* Brommer H, van Weeren PR, Brama PA, et al. Quantification and age-related distribution of articular cartilage degeneration in the equine fetlock joint. Equine Vet J 2003;35(7):699; with permission.)

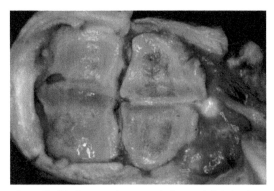

Fig. 2. End-stage osteoarthritis in a metacarpophalangeal joint, characterized by severe cartilage erosion. The synovial membrane is inflamed.

and pathophysiologic aspects of joint pain is necessary for a rational treatment of clinical OA.

Joint pain

There are 2 general types of pain stimuli in synovial joints: mechanical stimuli, originating from mechanical changes in the environment of the joint (eg, through direct trauma), and chemical stimuli caused by inflammation. In case of chronic OA, both mechanical alterations and inflammation are present, but most of the pain is generated by the recurrent and intermittent inflammation that is triggered by the interaction of tissue damage and mechanical loading. These stimuli are detected and forwarded by different mechanoreceptors and nociceptors and the signal is then forwarded by Aδ or C-nerve fibers in peripheral nerves to the dorsal horn of the spinal cord. In the dorsal horn, neuromodulators and neurotransmitters are located within synapses between primary and secondary neurons. These secondary neurons run via the spinal cord to the brain where the signal is modulated and perceived.[20]

Nociception in the joint

Articular cartilage is aneural, but all other constituting elements of the joint are innervated and some of them very richly. In joints, 4 types of afferent receptors can be discerned.[21] The type 1 receptors are low-threshold mechanoreceptors that are connected to medium-sized myelinated nerve fibers and principally have a proprioceptive function. They are located in the joint capsule, but not in the synovial membrane. Type 2 receptors are large encapsulated end organs connected to myelinated nerve fibers that function as low-threshold mechanoreceptors and are typically found at the junction of the fibrous joint capsule and the subsynovial adipose tissue. They are activated only when the joint is in motion and act as dynamic proprioceptive sensors. Type 3 receptors are relatively large, thinly encapsulated end organs that are located close to the bony insertions of intraarticular and periarticular ligaments. Their threshold is high and they are only activated when joint motion reaches its physiologic limits. They are both mechanoreceptive and nociceptive, are connected to very rapidly conducing myelinated fibers, and act as safety mechanisms. Receptors of type 4 receptors consist of free nerve endings of afferent nonmyelinated C-fibers or small myelinated Aδ fibers. They are widely distributed over the entire joint capsule including the synovial membrane. They are also abundant in the periosteum directly adjacent to the joint margins. These receptors have a high threshold and respond to thermal, chemical, and mechanical stimuli. Chemical stimuli provoked by inflammation may increase their responsiveness to mechanical stimuli and thus lead to sensitization of the joint, thereby causing hyperalgesia and/or allodynia.

Sources of joint pain in osteoarthritis

In OA, there are numerous interacting processes that can contribute to the perception of joint pain and it is rare that a single, precise tissue origin of pain can be identified in the individual patient (**Fig. 3**). Depending on individual disease stage, the fluctuating degree of inflammation and activity of the patient, the richly innervated subchondral bone, marginal periosteum, synovial membrane and joint capsule will all, to a variable extent, contribute to pain and loss of function in OA. In human medicine, it is generally accepted that there is no straightforward relationship between tissue damage and pain level.[18] In human OA patients, alterations of central nervous system pathways associated with chronic pain (central sensitization) have been identified. This phenomenon may, to a certain extent, explain the difficulties encountered in long-term management of OA pain.[22] It is not known whether this plays a role in the horse as well. Synovitis is an important factor in OA because it contributes to pain through joint effusion, swelling, and/or fibrosis, leading to activation of mechanoreceptors in the joint capsule and direct chemical stimulation of nociceptors.

Management of Chronic Joint Disease in the Geriatric Horse

There is no therapy that succeeds in the regeneration of hyaline cartilage once substantial damage to the articular cartilage layer has occurred and the famous statement from William Hunter (1743) that "ulcerated cartilage when destroyed is never recovered" (**Fig. 4**)[23] still stands, despite great efforts in biomedical research (**Box 1**). This applies to young and middle-aged individuals, but obviously more so

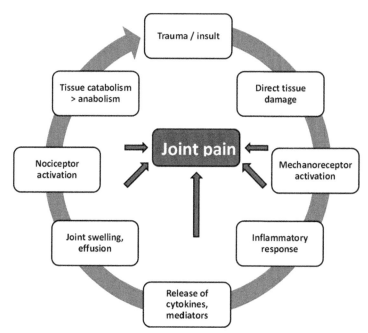

Fig. 3. Simplified scheme representing processes that may lead to joint pain in the vicious cycle of events occurring in osteoarthritis. (*From* van Weeren PR, de Grauw JC. Pain in osteoarthritis. Vet Clin North Am Equine Pract 2010;26:624; with permission.)

> If we confult the ftandard Chirurgical Writers from *Hippocrates* down to the prefent Age, we fhall find, that an ulcerated Cartilage is univerfally allowed to be a very troublefome Difeafe; that it admits of a Cure with more Difficulty than a carious Bone; and that, when deftroyed, it is never recovered.

Fig. 4. Facsimile reproduction of the original text by William Hunter as published in the *Philosophic Transactions of the Royal Society of London* in 1743.

to geriatric patients in whom the disease is more advanced. The aim of treatment is, however, different in the latter category. In the performance horse, therapeutic efforts will focus on bringing the animal back in competition as soon as possible and doping issues may be relevant. In geriatric horses, the aim is to reach a sustainable and preferably steady condition in which the horse is as comfortable as possible and doping is not an issue. These factors will influence the choice of treatment. Treatment may consist of local treatment of the affected joint(s), pain management, and supportive treatments such as farriery, physiotherapy, and exercise management, and is often a combination of these. Another important aspect of the management of chronic joint disease is the exercise regimen that is applied.

Local treatment of osteoarthritis in the elderly horse
The choice of possible intraarticular treatments of OA has increased considerably over the past decade with the advent of biologic therapies consisting of either (stem) cells or cellular products, such as platelet-rich plasma and autologous conditioned serum. For recent overviews, see Frisbie 2016.[24,25] There is some preliminary and/or anecdotal evidence that some of these treatments may be beneficial and, although any data are lacking, there is no known reason why they could in principle not be applied to geriatric horses. However, these therapies are meant to be disease modifying in active performance horses rather than palliative, and are expensive. This makes them certainly not first-choice treatments in geriatric horses with end-stage disease and they will not be considered further in this text, limiting intraarticular treatment options to corticosteroids and some other drugs such as hyaluronan and polysulfated glycosaminoglycans (PSGAGs).

The principal use of corticosteroids in OA is the rapid treatment of the intermittently occurring flares. Untreated, the effects of flares may linger on for a prolonged period,

---

Box 1
Principles of management of chronic joint disease in the geriatric horse

- Treat every flare-up directly (in severe cases, short- or medium-acting corticosteroids; pain management through systemic nonsteroidal antiinflammatory drugs).
- Reduce weight, if obese.
- Optimize housing conditions, and soft surfaces.
- Consider specific orthopedic shoeing.
- Improve or maintain joint stability and balance as much as possible through controlled exercise.

because the inflammation will only fade slowly. This prolonged inflammation leads to long periods of disturbed joint homeostasis and hence to further deterioration of the already affected articular tissues, rendering them more vulnerable for a next event. Immediate treatment with a potent antiinflammatory drug such as a corticosteroid in case of severe flares will not only lead to the animal becoming more comfortable, but also limit the aggravation of the existing damage. Several corticosteroids are available for clinical use (**Table 1**). Of these, the use of methylprednisolone acetate is currently discouraged because of deleterious side effects, whereas no such effects have been reported for betamethasone or triamcinolone acetonide, which have even been shown to be chondroprotective.[26] The chance of development of laminitis, which traditionally has been associated with the use of intraarticular corticosteroids and certainly would be a concern in the elderly horse, has been shown to be very limited. A study from the 1980s showed no laminitis in 1200 horses treated with triamcinolone acetonide at a maximal dose of 18 mg[27] and in a more recent study only 3 cases were seen in 2000 horses, many of which were treated with higher doses.[28] Therefore, there is no basis for discouraging the judicious use of intraarticular corticosteroids in case of serious flares of OA.

Hyaluronan (hyaluronic acid [HA]) and PSGAG are widely used in the treatment of equine OA. In a recent survey among 831 equine practitioners more than 50% used regular injections of HA to treat chronic cases of OA, also if there were radiographic changes, that is, in advanced stages of the disease.[29] PGAGs were also frequently used (in almost 60% of chronic cases and in just <50% of cases with radiographic evidence), but here the intramuscular application was generally chosen, not the intraarticular route. Both drugs claim to be both symptom-modifying (ie, palliative) and disease modifying (ie, to a certain extent curative), for which claims there is better evidence for PSGAGs than for HA.[30,31] Although not much can be expected from any disease-modifying action in advanced OA in geriatric horses, there are also no contraindications to use these products in this population, apart from increased costs.

Systemic treatment of osteoarthritis in the elderly horse

Pain is the most important clinical feature of OA with the greatest impact on both welfare and performance. The recurrent lameness episodes that are emblematic for OA in the horse are manifestations of pain. There are 2 important issues that should be considered and that are of greater concern in pain management in geriatric horses

Table 1
Overview of the most commonly used corticosteroids for intraarticular use in the horse

Name of the Drug	Duration of Action	Dosage (mg)	Remarks
Methylprednisolone acetate	Long	40–100	The lower end of the dosage range is recommended for an optimal effect while avoiding damage at a longer term
Betamethasone acetate	Medium to long	3–18	—
Triamcinolone acetonide	Medium	6–18	Most commonly used

From van Weeren PR, de Grauw JC. Pain in osteoarthritis. Vet Clin North Am Equine Pract 2010;26:630; with permission.

with end-stage OA than in younger animals featuring less joint damage. First, pain treatment is palliative and does not treat the underlying disease process (but still may have its influence on that process). Second, prolonged and often even life-long treatment may be necessary, making possible side effects as well as cost aspects very relevant.

Nonsteroidal antiinflammatory drugs (NSAIDs) form by far the most important category of drugs used for the treatment of musculoskeletal pain. These drugs inhibit the enzyme cyclooxygenase (COX) in the arachidonic acid cascade, thus affecting prostaglandin production. Of the isoenzymes COX-1 and COX-2, COX-1 exerts physiologic functions such as the protection of mucosal barriers in the gastrointestinal tract and the latter is more inflammation related. For this reason, selective COX-2 inhibitors have been developed as opposed to the older generation of general COX inhibitors. Selective COX-2 inhibitors have also become available for the treatment of OA in the horse, but older generation nonselective NSAIDs are still widely used, with phenylbutazone (PBZ) as most prominent example (**Table 2**).

PBZ, or "bute," has been used in horses for more than 50 years and is still the most widely used drug in equine orthopedic practice, in which it is seen as the most cost-effective treatment for OA pain.[32] In human medicine, the drug is no longer approved in many countries because of its association with a (slightly) increased risk of aplastic anemia.[33] For the same reason, the drug has been withheld registration for equine use in some countries. PBZ is typically used orally in a dose of 2.2 mg/kg twice a day (BID) or tapered to once a day (QD) after an initial loading dose of 4.4 mg/kg BID over 2 days. The drug is generally seen as very effective in musculoskeletal pain by equine practitioners. Recent in vivo research has shown that at joint level the drug does not limit inflammation-induced cartilage catabolism and may reduce collagen anabolism

Table 2
Overview of the most commonly used NSAIDs with their route of administration and dosage

Name of the Drug	Application	Dosage	Remarks
Phenylbutazone	Oral	2.2 mg/kg BID (initial loading dose often 4.4 mg/kg for 2 d and in case of long-term use standard dose tapered to QD)	Use in some countries not authorized because of perceived human health risk
Flunixin	Oral/IV	1.1 mg/kg QD	—
Carprofen	IV/oral	0.7 mg/kg (IV) QD 1.4 mg/kg (oral) QD	—
Ketoprofen	IV/IM	2.2 mg/kg QD	In oral form not bioavailable
Vedaprofen	Oral	Initial dose 2 mg/kg BID, maintenance 1 mg/kg BID	—
Meloxicam	Oral	0.6 mg/kg QD	Only NSAID with shown positive effect on cartilage metabolism in vivo
Naproxen	Oral/IV	10 mg/kg BID or QD	—

Abbreviations: BID, twice a day; IM, intramuscular; IV, intravenous; NSADI, nonsteroidal antiinflammatory drug; QD, once a day.

From van Weeren PR, de Grauw JC. Pain in osteoarthritis. Vet Clin North Am Equine Pract 2010;26:627; with permission.

transiently as evidenced by Synovial fluid markers.[34] PBZ has a relatively narrow safety margin and may have severe toxic side effects when recommended dosages are exceeded, during prolonged treatment, and/or in susceptible animals (such as geriatric horses, ponies, foals, and animals with vascular, renal, or hepatic compromise[35]). The potentially lethal adverse effects include gastrointestinal ulceration, renal papillary necrosis, and thrombosis.

Flunixin is used most widely for the treatment of abdominal pain. It is, however, also effective for the alleviation of lameness[36] and was shown to be equally efficacious to PBZ in horses with navicular disease.[37] There are no in vivo data on possible effects of the drug on joint homeostasis. Flunixin is generally administered at a dose of 1.1 mg/kg QD orally or intravenously (IV). Toxicity is low; adverse effects became only apparent at 5 times the recommended daily dose.[38]

Carprofen is a relatively potent analgesic in horses that is administered at 0.7 mg/kg IV or orally at a dose of 1.4 mg/kg. Several in vitro studies have suggested positive effects on joint homeostasis,[39,40] but no in vivo data exist for horses. Carprofen has a relatively narrow therapeutic index; adverse effects may develop at twice the recommended dose.[41]

Ketoprofen has been shown to accumulate in inflamed tissues, but was found to be inferior to PBZ in treating acute joint inflammation in a synovitis model.[42] The recommended dose of is 2.2 mg/kg IV QD. It is a safe drug, but has as its main disadvantage that it is not orally bioavailable, precluding routine use in chronic joint disease.

Vedaprofen has been registered for oral use (initial dose 2 mg/kg BID, maintenance 1 mg/kg BID) in several countries. Vedaprofen seems to have more affinity for COX-1 than COX-2.[43] Nothing is known about its effects on the primary process of OA. The clinical impression exists that the analgesic efficacy of vedaprofen for orthopedic pain compares unfavorably with PBZ, which may explain the fact that in countries where the use of PBZ is either illegal or restricted meloxicam rather than vedaprofen is the preferred oral NSAID for orthopedic diseases.

Meloxicam (orally dosed at 0.6 mg/kg QD) is a potent antiinflammatory and analgesic drug. Meloxicam was also the most selective COX-2 inhibitor of 4 examined NSAIDs (with PBZ, flunixin, and carprofen).[44] Meloxicam is the only NSAID for which evidence exists for favorable in vivo effects on cartilage metabolism. In a lipopolysaccharide-induced arthritis, model meloxicam was able to mitigate the catabolic effects of acute joint inflammation on articular cartilage.[45] However, it remains to be seen whether this is also true for chondroprotection in the longer term.

Naproxen is rarely used for the alleviation of equine musculoskeletal pain, but was proven more potent than PBZ in an equine myositis model[46] and has a wide safety margin. It is administered orally or IV at a dose of 10 mg/kg BID or QD.

Some other systemically administered OA drugs, such as IV applied HA and intramuscular PSGAGs (see above) also provide analgesia to some extent, but this is secondary to their influence on the primary disease process. They are not generally used for their analgesic effect in OA and there is no *rationale* for their use to this end in geriatric horses suffering from end-stage disease.

New developments in pain control of chronic joint disease
Pain medication in chronic joint disease often has to be administered over prolonged periods. Many, if not all, of the NSAIDs may produce severe side effects if used in this way. This is a big problem in human medicine and, together with the fact that OA is

mostly restricted to a limited number of joints, it has prompted the quest for local delivery systems that permit the controlled release of medication in the joint cavity. The obvious advantage is that much lower doses are necessary than in case of systemic application, thus avoiding undesired side effects. Some of these systems have been tested in the horse with promising preliminary results. Larsen and colleagues[47] reported the injection into equine carpal joints of 2 mL in situ forming depot composed of polyethylene glycol and the NSAID celecoxib loaded at 290 mg celecoxib per gram of solution. They reported low concentrations (less than the detection level of approximately 1 ng/mL) of celecoxib in serum samples for 10 days after intraarticular administration, but did not report synovial fluid concentrations. In another study the intraarticular tolerability and suitability for local and sustained release of an in situ forming polymer-based gel, loaded with 2 dosages of celecoxib, 50 mg/g ('low celecoxib gel') and 260 mg/g ('high celecoxib gel') was investigated in horse joints.[48] In the synovial fluid, concentrations of celecoxib were detected until 4 weeks after administration (**Fig. 5**). Celecoxib was also detected in plasma, but peaked at very low concentrations (150 ng/mL) and was detectable until day 3 after administration, after which its concentration was less than the detection limit. Controlled intraarticular release using either gel or nanoparticle technology seems promising therefore, especially for use in geriatric horses in which liver function may be compromised and where doping issues normally are not relevant.

Nutraceuticals

Feed additives or nutraceuticals are used at a very large scale worldwide and many of them claim to be beneficial for (chronic) joint disease. Many of these supplements contain glucosamine and/or chondroitin sulfate, both natural components of articular cartilage, with or without addition of a large variety of other compounds. For a recent overview see McIlwraith (2016).[49] The evidence for in vivo efficacy remains very thin,

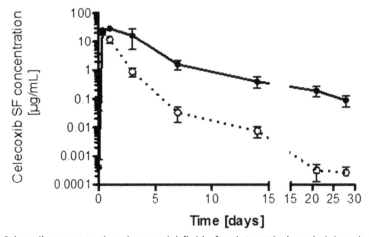

Fig. 5. Celecoxib concentrations in synovial fluid after intraarticular administration in the talocrural joint of a polymer-based gel, loaded with 2 dosages of celecoxib (CLB), 50 mg/g ('low CLB gel', *open circles*) and 260 mg/g ('high CLB gel', *closed circles*). The high dose retained a concentration of greater than 100 ng/mL for more than 4 weeks. In serum the concentration had fallen to less than 50 ng/mL within 3 days and became undetectable shortly after (data not shown). (*From* Petit A, Redout EM, van de Lest CH, et al. Sustained intraarticular release of celecoxib from in situ forming gels made of acetyl-capped PCLA-PEG-PCLA triblock copolymers in horses. Biomaterials 2015;53:434; with permission.)

but a number of studies have shown a (limited) beneficial effect of some products. In a study on the effect of supplementation with extract from green-lipped mussels (*Perna canaliculus*) in 26 horses with primary fetlock lameness, subjective lameness parameters improved in treated horses versus placebo-treated animals.[50] In a study on the effects of avocado and soybean unsaponified extracts in experimentally induced joint disease, no clinical effect on lameness was seen, but the histologic appearance of the treated joints was better.[51] In the only study focusing specifically on geriatric horses (age 29 ± 4 years) in which kinematic outcome criteria were used to test the effect of a compound containing glucosamine, chondroitin sulfate and methyl sulfonyl methane, no effect on gait parameters was found and the claim that the product would improve stiff gait in elderly horses could hence not be substantiated.[52] Whereas joint supplements will not do harm and some of them may have a certain benefit; their cost-effectiveness ratio can be questioned.

Surgical Treatment

Various surgical interventions have been described for the treatment of heavily osteoarthritic joints that are beyond the stage that any intrinsic repair can still be expected and for which palliative treatment is insufficient to create an acceptable state of comfort for the animal. It can be questioned to what extent application of these mostly very invasive procedures in geriatric patients is ethically acceptable. Further, the application of major surgery to patients that have a reduced life expectancy will likely to be economically viable for only very valuable animals. For these reasons, surgical options are not discussed further in this context.

Supportive Treatments

There are various options for supportive treatments and management procedures for the treatment of OA in the geriatric horse in addition to the pharmaceutical approach of flare-ups and pain management.

Repeated mechanical overloading is a well-known cause of OA. Two factors are important here: the number of repeats and the intensity of loading. The most important determining factor of the latter is the impact peak just after the hoof hits the ground with the high deceleration at that moment creating severe impact vibrations that put heavy stress on the tissues of the lower limb. This impact peak is determined by both the surface and the hoof and can be influenced by shoeing. Impact vibrations have been shown to be 15% less in unshod hooves compared with steel-shod hooves.[53] In some cases, leaving horses unshod may not be an option and for those cases various types of rims between the hoof wall and the shoes or padding of the sole have been developed that may dampen impact vibrations significantly[54] and that can be used to make the horse affected by chronic degenerative joint disease more comfortable.[55]

Optimization of joint stability and proprioception is important to prevent aberrant loading of joints. This is of special importance in geriatric patients, because neuromuscular changes associated with aging are known to manifest as a decrease in strength and coordination preceding a loss in muscle mass.[56] There are various physiotherapy techniques that aim at improving muscular fitness, strength, and coordination.[57,58] Controlled exercise may play a role here too, but care should be taken to ensure that the surface is even and horses should not be forced to exercise during flare-ups of joint disease. To prevent aggravation of chronic OA, care should be taken that exercise is discontinued when signs of fatigue become apparent, because fatigue-induced incoordination may lead to increased joint instability. Manual flexing exercises to improve joint range of motion can be carried out, but are laborious and are of little benefit in elderly horses with end-stage disease. Low-grade continuous (pasture) exercise is more efficient in such cases.

Obese horses should lose weight, not only to reduce mechanical loading of the articulations, but also to decrease the low-grade inflammation that is a consequence of the systemic inflammatory load caused by cytokine production from adipose tissue, which is known to be an important etiologic factor of OA in humans.[59] It is not known whether a similar mechanism exists in the horse, but it has been demonstrated in small rodents, so it is likely that this is the case. Obesity is a widespread, although still insufficiently perceived problem in horses.[60] Additional measures that can be taken in the management of the geriatric horse with OA are supplying well-protected stabling of sufficient size to get up and lie down easily, providing good and dry bedding and, where possible, avoiding damp and cold weather.

CHRONIC LAMINITIS AND HOOF CARE OF THE GERIATRIC HORSE
Pathogenic Mechanisms

The etiology of laminitis is complex and will not be dealt with in detail in this context, but there is consensus that the main causal factors are inflammatory toxins, mechanical overloading, or metabolic and endocrine influences.[61] Underlying endocrinopathy may play an important and hitherto underestimated role in laminitis. Evidence of endocrinopathy was present in 89% of horses in a hospital in Finland. Of these horses, one-third had a diagnosis of pituitary pars intermedia dysfunction (PPID), and two-thirds showed basal hyperinsulinemia indicative of insulin resistance, without evidence of hirsutism.[62] In another study, the prevalence of PPID as defined by high plasma adrenocorticotropic hormone concentration in a single sample was 70% in a cohort of laminitic horses.[63] The suggested pathogenic pathway is a dysfunction of the brain resulting in a shortage in dopamine release from the hypothalamus. This shortage induces an increase in the release of adrenocorticotropic hormone and other peptides from the hypophysis, ultimately resulting in insulin resistance, higher insulin levels, and vascular constriction.[64]

There are several pathogenic pathways of laminitis, but all lead to structural failure of the attachments between the horny hoof capsule to the third phalanx, which is called the suspensory apparatus of the distal phalanx.[65] Bypass of the blood circulation in the hoof wall by vascular anastomosis with ischemia of the primary and secondary lamellae is one of these pathways.[66]

At older ages and thus in geriatric horses the chance of developing lameness owing to laminitis increases significantly.[67] In principle, all causal factors may play a role in the geriatric horse as in the nongeriatric horse, but endocrine disorders are more prevalent in geriatric horses than in younger ones. Pituitary dysfunction is the most common specific post mortem diagnosis in older horses.[68] In the study by Karikoski and colleagues,[62] horses with laminitis associated with an underlying endocrinopathy were significantly older and more likely to be pony breeds than the general nonlaminitic hospital population during the same period.

Treatment Considerations

The ultimate goal of treatment in geriatric horses, for whom performance is generally no longer a major consideration, is to attain a stable situation that will have the least possible impact on equine welfare (**Box 2**). Fatal progression of disease (**Fig. 6**) has to be avoided at all cost. This implies first of all treatment of the primary cause. In cases of PPID, treatment with pergolide has been reported to lead to significant improvement in clinical signs.[69] Pain management using NSAIDs (see above) is

---

Box 2
Principles of management of laminitis in the geriatric horse

- Treat every flare-up directly, that is, pain management through systemic nonsteroidal antiinflammatory drugs, first week: full dose, then half dose or every other day.
- Treat primary cause: pergolide.
- Adjust diet: remove concentrates, fresh grass and silage. Provide only hay (plus vitamin and mineral supplement).
- Take off shoes (if possible).
- Reduce toe length and rasp dorsal hoof wall.
- Apply wet hoof bandages every 2 days for a total of 4 days or put on wet shavings at the feeding location in combination with thick, soft stall bedding for lying down.
- Antiinflammatory/nonsteroidal antiinflammatory drugs: systemic, until 1 week after the horse has been shod.
- Vasodilation: acepromazine, until the horse is shod.
- Antithrombotic: calcium carbasalate, until 1 week after the horse has been shod.
- After improvement to Obel grade 2: apply open toe shoes with damping sole and firm hoof pad at the location of the frog.
- Start hand walking on a flat, soft surface three times a day.
- Repeat orthopedic shoeing at least once.
- Cold water on the feet more than 10 minutes each time twice a day depending on effect.

---

imperative, because laminitis is an extremely painful condition and, although inflammation in endocrine laminitis is less than with many other causes of the disorder,[70] some inflammation is occurring. The use of local anesthetics is not advised, because their use may lead to increased loading of the distal limb and more traction on the lamellae, with possibly fatal outcome. Food intake, especially of easily digestible carbohydrates, needs to be restricted and grain and concentrates should be withheld from the diet and replaced by good-quality hay.[71] To prevent microthrombosis in the hoof, the use of heparin, acetylsalicylic acid, or calcium carbasalate has been reported. Heparin would work prophylactically, but there are doubts regarding its clinical effectiveness.[72] Acepromazine is effective as a peripheral vasodilator and it increases the blood flow to the lamellae.[73] It can be applied orally or parenterally in low dosages, producing minimal sedative effects, although sedation can be beneficial because horses tend to lie down and thus relieve the pressure from their feet.[74] Glyceryl trinitrate pads have been applied locally, but there is no evidence for their effectiveness.[75]

Apart from the pharmaceutical treatment outlined, adaptations in the management of the horse with laminitis are crucial. The acutely laminitic horse needs to be strictly box rested to prevent further damage to the lamellae. Shoes must be removed at first instance and hooves need to be trimmed to distribute the forces exerted on the hoof as evenly as possible and thus to maximally reduce pressure. Maximal distribution of pressure together with an antiinflammatory effect can be achieved by putting the feet in wet bandages or stabling the horse on wet sand or soft bedding.[76] Wet bandages have the advantage that thick straw bedding can be provided for the horse to lay down comfortably.[71] Another option would be to have 1 part of the box filled with thick straw and the other part with wet sand where the horse eats its meals. Shortening the toe will facilitate break over and hence reduce the momentum on the site of attachment of the deep digital flexor tendon, reducing traction on the damaged lamellae.[77] In a

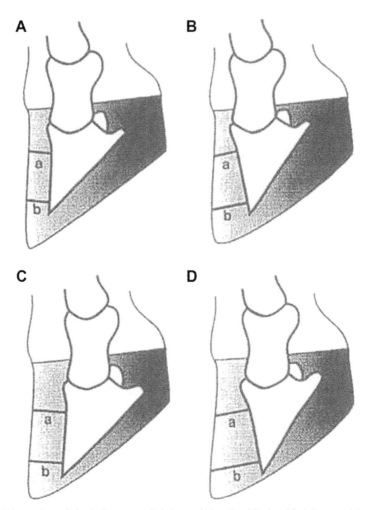

Fig. 6. Schematic radiologic Lateromedial view of the distal limb with (*A*) normal location of the third phalanx in the hoof capsule (a,b 19 ± 1 mm in warmbloods, 5° angle with the ground floor), (*B*) rotation, (*C*) sinker, and (*D*) rotation and sinker. (*From* Sloet van Oldruitenborgh-Oosterbaan MM. Laminitis in the horse: a review. Vet Q 1999;21(4):123; with permission.)

somewhat more chronic stage, a similar effect can be obtained by putting the horse on wedges.[78] Tenotomy of the flexor tendon is sometimes practiced, but should be considered a salvage procedure, because horses will not return to full athletic function.[79] Recently, research has started into the possible usefulness of *Clostridium botulinum* toxin type A as a muscle relaxant of the deep digital flexor muscle that may, either therapeutically or even preventively be used to reduce traction on the third phalanx in laminitis cases.[80,81]

For the more chronic situation, a large variety of shoes and frog supporting devices have been developed. Heart bar shoes can be purchased in an adjustable form.[82,83] The use of heart bar shoes has been shown to improve perfusion of the dorsal lamellae,[84] but substantial clinical improvement should not be expected during the first 7 days after therapeutic shoeing.[85] In our clinic, we advise open toe shoes at the time the horse allows lifting the feet (Obel grade 2). The palmar/plantar part of the feet is filled using a filler paste with a higher shore value to support the not painful and still well perfused frog.[86]

SUMMARY

As in humans, musculoskeletal disorders are the most prevalent health problem in aging horses. They are not life threatening, but are often painful and debilitating, and therefore are an important welfare issue. Chronic joint disease (OA) and chronic hoof problems (chronic laminitis) are the most prevalent single disorders. Treatment of OA in the elderly horse is basically similar to treatment of performance horses, but aims more at providing a stable situation with optimal comfort rather than at regaining the ability to compete. Immediate medical treatment of flare-ups, long-term pain management, and adaptation of (exercise) management and living conditions form the mainstay of treatment of OA in geriatric horses. Laminitis in the geriatric horse is related to pituitary dysfunction in many cases, which has an increased prevalence with age. Treatment of laminitis is basically similar to nongeriatric horses, but in PPID cases additional pergolide treatment has been shown to significantly improve clinical signs including a lameness/laminitis reduction for some time.

REFERENCES

1. Rossdale PD, Hopes R, Wingfield Digby NJ, et al. Epidemiological study of wastage among racehorses 1982 and 1983. Vet Rec 1985;116(3):66–9.
2. Olivier A, Nurton JP, Guthrie AJ. An epizoological study of wastage in thoroughbred racehorses in Gauteng, South Africa. J S Afr Vet Assoc 1997;68(4):125–9.
3. Bertuglia A, Bullone M, Rossotto F, et al. Epidemiology of musculoskeletal injuries in a population of harness Standardbred racehorses in training. BMC Vet Res 2014;10:11.
4. Reed SR, Jackson BF, McIlwraith CW, et al. Descriptive epidemiology of joint injuries in Thoroughbred racehorses in training. Equine Vet J 2012;44(1):13–9.
5. Egenvall A, Tranquille CA, Lönnell AC, et al. Days-lost to training and competition in relation to workload in 263 elite show-jumping horses in four European countries. Prev Vet Med 2013;112(3–4):387–400.
6. Jönsson L, Roepstorff L, Egenvall A, et al. Prevalence of clinical findings at examinations of young Swedish warmblood riding horses. Acta Vet Scand 2013;55:34.
7. Global Burden of Disease Study 2013 Collaborators. Global, regional, and national incidence, prevalence, and years lived with disability for 301 acute and chronic diseases and injuries in 188 countries, 1990-2013: a systematic analysis for the Global Burden of Disease Study 2013. Lancet 2015;386(9995):743–800.
8. Ireland JL, McGowan CM, Clegg PD, et al. A survey of health care and disease in geriatric horses aged 30 years or older. Vet J 2012;192(1):57–64.
9. Ireland JL, Clegg PD, McGowan CM, et al. Disease prevalence in geriatric horses in the United Kingdom: veterinary clinical assessment of 200 cases. Equine Vet J 2012;44(1):101–6.
10. Ireland JL, Clegg PD, McGowan CM, et al. Comparison of owner-reported health problems with veterinary assessment of geriatric horses in the United Kingdom. Equine Vet J 2012;44(1):94–100.
11. Ireland JL, Clegg PD, McGowan CM, et al. Factors associated with mortality of geriatric horses in the United Kingdom. Prev Vet Med 2011;101(3–4):204–18.
12. McIlwraith CW. Frank Milne lecture: from arthroscopy to gene therapy – 30 years of looking in joints. Proc Am Assoc Equine Pract 2005;51:65–113.

13. Radin EL, Rose RM. Role of subchondral bone in the initiation and progression of cartilage damage. Clin Orthop 1986;213:34–40.
14. Samuels J, Krasnokutsky S, Abramson SB. Osteoarthritis. A tale of three tissues. Bull NYU Hosp Joint Dis 2008;66(3):244–50.
15. Neundorf RH, Lowerison MB, Cruz AM, et al. Determination of the prevalence and severity of metacarpophalangeal joint osteoarthritis in Thoroughbred racehorses via quantitative macroscopic evaluation. Am J Vet Res 2010;71(11):1284–93.
16. Brommer H, van Weeren PR, Brama PA. New approach for quantitative assessment of articular cartilage degeneration in horses with osteoarthritis. Am J Vet Res 2003;64(1):83–7.
17. Brommer H, van Weeren PR, Brama PA, et al. Quantification and age-related distribution of articular cartilage degeneration in the equine fetlock joint. Equine Vet J 2003;35(7):697–701.
18. Perrot S. Osteoarthritis pain. Best Pract Res Clin Rheumatol 2015;29(1):90–7.
19. Goldring MB, Goldring SR. Osteoarthritis. J Cell Physiol 2007;213(3):626–34.
20. Raffa RB. Mechanism of action of analgesics used to treat osteoarthritis pain. Rheum Dis Clin North Am 2003;29:733–45.
21. van Weeren PR. General anatomy and physiology of joints. In: McIlwraith CW, Frisbie DD, Kawcak CE, et al, editors. Joint disease in the horse. 2nd edition. St Louis (MO): Elsevier; 2016. p. 1–24.
22. Gwilym SE, Keltner JR, Warnaby CE, et al. Psychophysical and functional imaging evidence supporting the presence of central sensitization in a cohort of osteoarthritis patients. Arthritis Rheum 2009;61(9):1226–34.
23. Hunter W. Of the structure and diseases of articulating cartilages. Proc R Soc Lond 1743;9:514–21.
24. Frisbie DD. Biologic therapies. In: McIlwraith CW, Frisbie DD, Kawcak CE, et al, editors. Joint disease in the horse. 2nd edition. St Louis (MO): Elsevier; 2016. p. 229–35.
25. Frisbie DD. Stem cells. In: McIlwraith CW, Frisbie DD, Kawcak CE, et al, editors. Joint disease in the horse. 2nd edition. St Louis (MO): Elsevier; 2016. p. 236–42.
26. McIlwraith CW. Intra-articular corticosteroids. In: McIlwraith CW, Frisbie DD, Kawcak CE, et al, editors. Joint disease in the horse. 2nd edition. St Louis (MO): Elsevier; 2016. p. 194–206.
27. Genovese RL. The use of corticosteroids in racetrack practice. In: Proc Symposium Effective Use of Corticosteroids in Veterinary Practice. Princeton, NJ: Veterinary Learning Systems; 1983. p. 56–65.
28. Bathe AP. The corticosteroid laminitis story: 3. The clinician's viewpoint. Equine Vet J 2007;39(1):7–11.
29. Ferris DJ, Frisbie DD, McIlwraith CW, et al. Current joint therapy usage in equine practice: a survey of veterinarians 2009. Equine Vet J 2011;43(5):530–5.
30. Frisbie DD. Hyaluronan. In: McIlwraith CW, Frisbie DD, Kawcak CE, et al, editors. Joint disease in the horse. 2nd edition. St Louis (MO): Elsevier; 2016. p. 215–9.
31. McIlwraith CW. Polysulfated glycosaminoglycan (Adequan®). In: McIlwraith CW, Frisbie DD, Kawcak CE, et al, editors. Joint disease in the horse. 2nd edition. St Louis (MO): Elsevier; 2016. p. 220–3.
32. Goodrich LR, Nixon AJ. Medical treatment of osteoarthritis in the horse – a review. Vet J 2006;171:51–69.
33. Risks of agranulocytosis and aplastic anemia. A first report of their relation to drug use with special reference to analgesics. The International Agranulocytosis and Aplastic Anemia Study. JAMA 1986;256:1749–57.

34. De Grauw JC, van Loon JP, van de Lest CH, et al. In vivo effects of phenylbuta-zone on inflammation and cartilage-derived biomarkers in equine joints with acute synovitis. Vet J 2014;201(1):51–6.
35. Owens JG, Clark TP. Analgesia. Vet Clin North Am Equine Pract 1999;15(3): 705–23.
36. Houdeshell JW, Hennessy PW. A new non-steroidal, anti-inflammatory analgesic for horses. J Equine Med Surg 1977;1:57–63.
37. Erkert RS, MacAllister CG, Payton ME, et al. Use of force plate analysis to compare the analgesic effects of intravenous administration of phenylbutazone and flunixin meglumine in horses with navicular syndrome. Am J Vet Res 2005; 66(2):284–8.
38. Trillo MA, Soto G, Gunson DE. Flunixin toxicity in a pony. Equine Pract 1984;6:21–9.
39. Frean SP, Abraham LA, Lees P. In vitro stimulation of equine articular cartilage proteoglycan synthesis by hyaluronan and carprofen. Res Vet Sci 1999;67: 183–90.
40. Armstrong S, Lees P. Effects of R and S enantiomers and a racemic mixture of carprofen on the production and release of proteoglycan and prostaglandin E2 from equine chondrocytes and cartilage explants. Am J Vet Res 1999;60:98–104.
41. May SA, Lees P. Nonsteroidal anti-inflammatory drugs. In: McIlwraith CW, Trotter GW, editors. Joint disease in the horse. Philadelphia: WB Saunders; 1996. p. 223–37.
42. Owens JG, Kamerling SG, Stanton SR, et al. Effects of pretreatment with ketopro-fen and phenylbutazone on experimentally induced synovitis in the horse. Am J Vet Res 1996;57:866–74.
43. Lees P, May SA, Hoeijmakers M, et al. A pharmacodynamic and pharmacokinetic study with vedaprofen in an equine model of acute nonimmune inflammation. J Vet Pharmacol Ther 1999;22:96–106.
44. Beretta C, Caravaglia G, Cavalli M. COX-1 and COX-2 inhibition in horse blood by phenylbutazone, flunixin, carprofen and meloxicam: an in vitro analysis. Pharma-col Res 2005;52:302–6.
45. De Grauw JC, van de Lest CHA, Brama PAJ, et al. In vivo effects of meloxicam on inflammatory mediators, MMP activity and cartilage biomarkers in equine joints with acute synovitis. Equine Vet J 2009;41:693–9.
46. Jones EW, Hamm D. Comparative efficacy of PBZ and naproxen in induced equine myositis. J Equine Med Surg 1978;2:341–7.
47. Larsen SW, Frost AB, Ostergaard J, et al. In vitro and in vivo characteristics of celecoxib in situ formed suspensions for intra-articular administration. J Pharm Sci 2011;100(10):4330–7.
48. Petit A, Redout EM, van de Lest CH, et al. Sustained intra-articular release of celecoxib from in situ forming gels made of acetyl-capped PCLA-PEG-PCLA triblock copolymers in horses. Biomaterials 2015;53:426–36.
49. McIlwraith CW. Use of oral joint supplements in equine joint disease. In: McIlwraith CW, Frisbie DD, Kawcak CE, et al, editors. Joint disease in the horse. 2nd edition. St Louis (MO): Elsevier; 2016. p. 277–80.
50. Cayzer J, Hedderley D, Gray S. A randomised, double-blinded, placebo-controlled study on the efficacy of a unique extract of green-lipped mussel (Perna canaliculus) in horses with chronic fetlock lameness attributed to osteoarthritis. Equine Vet J 2012;44(4):393–8.
51. Kawcak CE, Frisbie DD, McIlwraith CW, et al. Evaluation of avocado and soybean unsaponifiable extracts for treatment of horses with experimentally induced oste-oarthritis. Am J Vet Res 2007;68(6):598–604.

52. Higler MH, Brommer H, L'Ami JJ, et al. The effects of three-month oral supplementation with a nutraceutical and exercise on the locomotor pattern of aged horses. Equine Vet J 2014;46(5):611–7.
53. Willemen MA, Jacobs MW, Schamhardt HC. In vitro transmission and attenuation of impact vibrations in the distal forelimb. Equine Vet J Suppl 1999;30:245–8.
54. Benoit P, Barrey E, Regnault JC, et al. Comparison of the damping effect of different shoeing by the measurement of hoof acceleration. Acta Anat (Basel) 1993;146(2–3):109–13.
55. Back W, Pille F. The role of Hoof and Shoeing. In: Back W, Clayton HM, editors. Equine locomotion. 2nd edition. London: Elsevier; 2013. p. 147–74.
56. Hepple RT, Rice CL. Innervation and neuromuscular control in aging skeletal muscle. J Physiol 2015;594(8):1965–78.
57. Haussler KK. King MR physical rehabilitation. In: McIlwraith CW, Frisbie DD, Kawcak CE, et al, editors. Joint disease in the horse. 2nd edition. St Louis (MO): Elsevier; 2016. p. 243–69.
58. Stubbs N, Menke E, Back W, et al. Rehabilitation of the locomotor apparatus. In: Back W, Clayton HM, editors. Equine locomotion. 2nd edition. London: Elsevier; 2013. p. 381–417.
59. Roos EM, Arden NK. Strategies for the prevention of knee osteoarthritis. Nat Rev Rheumatol 2016;12(2):92–101.
60. Owers R, Chubbock S. Fight the fat! Equine Vet J 2013;45(1):5.
61. Katz LM, Bailey SR. A review of recent advances and current hypotheses on the pathogenesis of acute laminitis. Equine Vet J 2012;44:752–61.
62. Karikoski NP, Horn I, McGowan TW, et al. The prevalence of endocrinopathic laminitis among horses presented for laminitis at a first-opinion/referral equine hospital. Domest Anim Endocrinol 2011;41(3):111–7.
63. Donaldson MT, Jorgensen AJ, Beech J. Evaluation of suspected pituitary pars intermedia dysfunction in horses with laminitis. J Am Vet Med Assoc 2004;224:1123–7.
64. Gauff F, Patan-Zugaj B, Licka TF. Hyperinsulinaemia increases vascular resistance and endothelin-1 expression in the equine digit. Equine Vet J 2013;45(5):613–8.
65. van Eps AW. Acute laminitis: medical and supportive therapy. Vet Clin North Am Equine Pract 2010;26:103–14.
66. Hood DM, Grosenbaugh DA, Slater MR. Vascular perfusion in horses with chronic laminitis. Equine Vet J 1994;26(3):191–6.
67. Brosnahan MM, Paradis MR. Demographic and clinical characteristics of geriatric horses: 467 cases (1989-1999). J Am Vet Med Assoc 2003;223(1):93–8.
68. Miller MA, Moore GE, Bertin FR, et al. What's new in old horses? Postmortem diagnoses in mature and aged equids. Vet Pathol 2016;53(2):390–8.
69. Donaldson MT, LaMonte BH, Morresey P, et al. Treatment with pergolide or cyproheptadine of pituitary pars intermedia dysfunction (equine Cushing's disease). J Vet Intern Med 2002;16(6):742–6.
70. Karikoski NP, McGowan CM, Singer ER, et al. Pathology of natural cases of equine endocrinopathic laminitis associated with hyperinsulinemia. Vet Pathol 2015;52(5):945–56.
71. Sloet van Oldruitenborgh-Oosterbaan MM. Laminitis in the horse: a review. Vet Q 1999;21(4):121–7.
72. Moore BR, Hinchcliff KW. Heparin: a review of its pharmacology and therapeutic use in horses. J Vet Intern Med 1994;8(1):26–35.

73. Ingle-Fehr JE, Baxter GM. The effect of oral isoxsuprine and pentoxifylline on digital and laminar blood flow in healthy horses. Vet Surg 1999;28(3):154–60.
74. Wattle O, Ekfalck A, Funkquist B, et al. Behavioural studies in healthy ponies subjected to short-term forced recumbency aiming at an adjunctive treatment in an acute attack of laminitis. Zentralbl Veterinärmed A 1995;42(1):62–8.
75. Gilhooly MH, Eades SC, Stokes AM, et al. Effects of topical nitroglycerine patches and ointment on digital venous plasma nitric oxide concentrations and digital blood flow in healthy conscious horses. Vet Surg 2005;34(6):604–9.
76. van Eps AW, Pollitt CC. Equine laminitis: cryotherapy reduces the severity of the acute lesion. Equine Vet J 2004;36(3):255–60.
77. Baker WR Jr. Treating laminitis: beyond the mechanics of trimming and shoeing. Vet Clin North Am Equine Pract 2012;28(2):441–55.
78. McGuigan MP, Walsh TC, Pardoe CH, et al. Deep digital flexor tendon force and digital mechanics in normal ponies and ponies with rotation of the distal phalanx as a sequel to laminitis. Equine Vet J 2005;37(2):161–5.
79. Eastman TG, Honnas CM, Hague BA, et al. Deep digital flexor tenotomy as a treatment for chronic laminitis in horses: 35 cases (1988-1997). J Am Vet Med Assoc 1999;214(4):517–9.
80. Hardeman LC, van der Meij BR, Oosterlinck M, et al. Effect of Clostridium botulinum toxin type A injections into the deep digital flexor muscle on the range of motion of the metacarpus and carpus, and the force distribution underneath the hooves, of sound horses at the walk. Vet J 2013;198(Suppl 1):e152–6.
81. Wijnberg ID, Hardeman LC, van der Meij BR, et al. The effect of Clostridium botulinum toxin type A injections on motor unit activity of the deep digital flexor muscle in healthy sound Royal Dutch sport horses. Vet J 2013;198(Suppl 1):e147–51.
82. Eustace RA, Caldwell MN. The construction of the heart bar shoe and the technique of dorsal wall resection. Equine Vet J 1989;21(5):367–9.
83. Eustace RA, Caldwell MN. Treatment of solar prolapse using the heart bar shoe and dorsal hoof wall resection technique. Equine Vet J 1989;21(5):370–2.
84. Ritmeester AM, Blevins WE, Ferguson DW, et al. Digital perfusion, evaluated scintigraphically, and hoof wall growth in horses with chronic laminitis treated with egg bar-heart bar shoeing and coronary grooving. Equine Vet J Suppl 1998;26:111–8.
85. Taylor D, Hood DM, Wagner IP. Short-term effect of therapeutic shoeing on severity of lameness in horses with chronic laminitis. Am J Vet Res 2002;63(12):1629–33.
86. Olivier A, Wannenburg J, Gottschalk RD, et al. The effect of frog pressure and downward vertical load on hoof wall weight-bearing and third phalanx displacement in the horse–an in vitro study. J S Afr Vet Assoc 2001;72(4):217–27.

Ophthalmologic Disorders in Aged Horses

Fernando Malalana, DVM, FHEA, MRCVS

KEYWORDS

- Geriatric • Horse • Eye • Uveitis • Blind

KEY POINTS

- Ocular abnormalities are common in aged horses.
- Superficial nonhealing corneal ulcers seem more prevalent in older horses, perhaps as a result of decreased corneal sensitivity.
- Significant ocular disorder as a result of recurrent uveitis can manifest more clearly as horses age. Important consequences of recurrent uveitis are cataracts and glaucoma.
- Several retinal and vitreal abnormalities are commonly seen in old horses, with variable effects on vision.

INTRODUCTION

Ophthalmologic disease seems to be common in geriatric animals. Analysis of the records of a large number of geriatric ($\geq$20 years old) horses admitted to an American veterinary hospital indicated that 11% had ocular disease.[1] However, this prevalence increased when the general equine geriatric population was considered. Studies in the United Kingdom have shown that 94% of horses 15 years of age or older had at least 1 ocular abnormality detected by a veterinarian.[2–4] This number increased to 100% when only horses 30 years of age or older were examined.[5] Only approximately 3.5% of owners reported any ocular problems in these horses, and 10% noted ocular discharge. Survey studies in Australia have also shown a high prevalence of ocular disease; 22.3% of horses 15 years of age and older in Queensland were reported to have ocular discharge, making this the fourth most common clinical sign mentioned by owners.[6] A clear positive correlation was noted between the presence of ocular discharge and increasing age. Again, although ocular discharge seemed to be common, only 3.3% of owners reported ocular problems in their horses and only 2.6% perceived eyesight as an important health issue. It seems that a large number of aged horses may have undetected ocular disease that could be a source of chronic

Conflicts of Interest: The author declares no conflicts of interest.
Philip Leverhulme Equine Hospital, University of Liverpool, Leahurst Campus, Chester High Road, Neston CH64 7TE, UK
E-mail address: f.malalana@liverpool.ac.uk

low-grade discomfort. In addition, some of these ophthalmic abnormalities may have a significant effect on the horses' vision, with important human safety and animal welfare implications. This article reviews the most common ocular abnormalities in geriatric horses.

CORNEAL DISEASE

Corneal disease is a common problem in equine practice.[7] In a study assessing the prevalence of disease in a geriatric (≥15 years old) population, corneal lesions were detected in 2.6% of the horses examined.[3] These abnormalities included corneal edema, opacities, and scarring.

As part of the aging process, changes occur that affect the ocular surface. In humans, the lacrimal gland has been shown to decrease its secretion with age.[8] Tear deficiency and evaporative dry eye syndromes are rare in horses,[9] but these may become more common with increasing age.[10] Although studies have shown no difference in the amount of tear production between young and old horses,[11] orbital fat loss may result in enophthalmos and inadequate spreading and stability of the tear film.[10] In addition, the composition of the tear film also varies. The levels of lactoferrin and lysozyme, two potent antimicrobial agents, have been shown to decrease with age.[8,12] Other factors can also influence the immune response on the ocular surface in older animals, such as a reduced phagocytic activity of polymorphonuclear leukocytes and impaired T-cell function.[12] This combination of factors can increase the susceptibility to microbial disease, especially keratomycosis, and may make these conditions more difficult to treat as horses get older. For these reasons, it may be advisable to select bactericidal rather than bacteriostatic antimicrobials when treating bacterial keratitis. In addition, topical corticosteroids should be used with caution where these are warranted for ocular conditions.[12]

Superficial ulcerative keratitis is one of the most commonly observed ophthalmic problems in horses. In most cases the ulceration heals without complications in 24 to 72 hours[13]; however, on some occasions these ulcers show a prolonged healing time or fail to epithelize. These superficial, nonhealing corneal ulcers are characterized by the presence of chronic (>1 week) ulceration with redundant, loose epithelial borders and no evidence of stromal involvement, infectious agents, or inflammatory cellular infiltrate[7,13–15] (Fig. 1). Superficial nonhealing corneal ulcers can

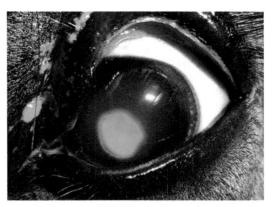

Fig. 1. Superficial, nonhealing, corneal ulcer in a 15-year-old mare. Note the poorly defined ulcer margins and the underrunning of fluorescein beyond the edge of the ulcer, indicating poorly adhered epithelium.

affect horses of any age but they seem to be more common in middle-aged to aged patients.[7,13,14] The reason for this increased prevalence as horses get older is probably multifactorial. Keratocyte density seems to be higher in younger individuals than in adults[16] and there is also thickening of the epithelial basement membrane with age,[8] which may contribute to the delayed healing. Perhaps more importantly there is a decrease in the nerve density at the level of the sub-basal plexus, below the epithelium.[8] The cornea is the most densely innervated tissue of the body, and these nerve fibers exert trophic influences on the corneal epithelium, stimulating the growth, proliferation, and differentiation of the epithelial cells and the production of type VII collagen.[11] Reduction in corneal sensitivity can result in epithelial defects and ulceration. Studies assessing the corneal touch threshold with a Cochet-Bonnet esthesiometer showed a significant decrease in corneal sensitivity between young (<10 years) and old (>15 years) horses, and this decrease was more marked if the older horses were showing clinical signs of pituitary pars intermedia dysfunction.[11]

Superficial, nonhealing corneal ulcers can represent a clinical challenge and numerous surgical treatment options are commonly required, such as debridement of the elevated epithelial edges manually or with a diamond burr, punctate or grid keratotomy, and/or superficial keratectomy with or without conjunctival flaps.[7,13,14] Anecdotally, some cases seem to respond better to treatment when serum from a young horse is applied topically on the ocular surface.[10]

With aging there is also a decrease in the number and density of corneal endothelial cells.[8,16] These cells are essential for maintaining the dehydrated status of the cornea. Animals are born with a fixed number of corneal endothelial cells, and this number decreases gradually with age. Because these cells do not divide, cell loss induced by age or disease cannot be reversed. This cell loss leads to corneal edema and loss of corneal transparency. In addition, this accumulation of fluid can induce the separation of the corneal epithelium from the underlying stroma in the form of small blisters known as bullae[8] that may also affect ulcer healing. Primary corneal endothelial dystrophy has been reported as a cause of age-related corneal edema in horses, frequently presenting clinically as a central vertical band[17] (**Fig. 2**). This condition should be differentiated from other potential causes of corneal edema, such as glaucoma, uveitis, or traumatic injury.[10]

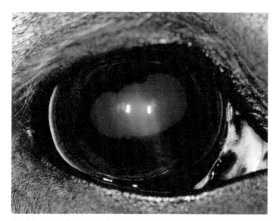

Fig. 2. Central, vertical band of corneal edema in an otherwise normal eye of a 19-year-old warmblood gelding. Serial measurements of the intraocular pressure have always remained within normal limits.

UVEITIS

Equine recurrent uveitis (ERU) is a spontaneous disease characterized by repeated episodes of intraocular inflammation.[18] Although a uveitic episode can occur at any age, a clear correlation ($r = 0.983$) has been found between age and the occurrence of ERU.[19] One study in the United Kingdom found uveal abnormalities in 23.4% of horses 15 years of age and older,[3] although another study in Germany detected signs of ERU in almost a third of horses from the same age group. In the United States, the mean age at presentation for ERU was 11.6 and 13.3 years depending on whether the horses were seropositive or seronegative to *Leptospira* spp respectively.[20] Signs of acute anterior uveitis include ocular pain, blepharospasm, lacrimation, chemosis, corneal changes (including edema, vascularization, and keratic precipitates), aqueous flare, hypopyon, hyphema, marked miosis, and iris color changes. Posterior uveitis can be more difficult to diagnose and is characterized by vitritis with liquefaction of the vitreous, vitreal floaters, and retinal changes. Because of the recurrent nature of the disease, changes associated with previous episodes are sometimes noted in an otherwise quiescent eye; these include corneal scarring, iris depigmentation, synechiae, granula iridica degeneration, cataracts, glaucoma, phthisis bulbi, and fundic changes[10,21] (**Fig. 3**).

In geriatric horses with ERU, because of the potential for a lifetime of accumulated episodes of intraocular inflammation, significant ocular disorder is commonly observed. Secondary complications such as cataracts and glaucoma are frequent (see elsewhere in the text) and vision can be significantly affected. Frequently in these cases treatment is directed to avoid further deterioration and control the painful episodes. Suprachoroid slow-release cyclosporine A implants have been successfully used in patients with ERU to provide long-term control of the condition.[22] Enucleation may be indicated for blind eyes in which the painful episodes cannot be avoided.

GLAUCOMA

Although the estimated prevalence of glaucoma in the general equine population is considered low, geriatric horses are at increased risk, with a recent study documenting that 65% of glaucoma cases presented in horses older than 15 years.[23–29] There

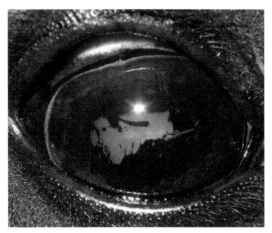

Fig. 3. An 18-year-old Welsh section D gelding showing signs of chronic intraocular inflammation in his right eye. Note the abnormal superior limbal margin, ruptured granula iridica, abnormal pupillary margin with numerous synechiae and dense cataract.

are 2 routes by which the aqueous humor exits the eye: the conventional and the un-conventional pathways.[25–29] The conventional pathway refers to aqueous outflow via the iridocorneal angle and trabecular meshwork. With age, the trabecular meshwork changes histologically: the trabecular endothelial cellularity is reduced and the outflow spaces are decreased, which may account for an increase in intraocular pressure observed in older horses.[16] The unconventional pathway makes reference to the drainage of fluid via the uveoscleral route. An age-related decrease in intracellular pores in the scleral venous sinus has been shown, which may also result in a decrease in aqueous flow facility.[16] However, age alone may not explain the increased risk of glaucoma in geriatric horses. Most cases of equine glaucoma are secondary to ERU, in which the deposition of inflammatory cells and debris at the drainage angle and the presence of adhesions and inflammatory fibrovascular membranes affect and limit the outflow of aqueous humor.[24]

Horses seem to tolerate higher intraocular pressures for longer compared with dogs or humans.[24,26–28] In addition, clinical signs of glaucoma in horses tend to be subtle, with little evidence of ocular discomfort, making diagnosis difficult. Signs commonly associated with glaucoma in horses include hydrophthalmos, corneal edema, corneal striae (Haab striae), a mildly dilated pupil, lens luxation, and optic nerve cupping and degeneration (**Fig. 4**). Signs of chronic intraocular inflammation are frequently observed in cases secondary to ERU. The intraocular pressure shows diurnal variation in horses, so, if glaucoma is suspected, repeat measurement may be required.[24–29] Pressures more than 30 mm Hg indicate glaucoma. It is important that, when repeat measurements are taken, these are done in identical circumstances; factors such as head positioning, placement of an auriculopalpebral nerve block, or sedation can greatly affect the measurements.[26,28,30,31]

Medical therapy for glaucoma involves the administration of drugs that reduce aqueous humor production. β-Blockers, such as 0.5% timolol maleate, and carbonic anhydrase inhibitors, such as 2% dorzolamide or 1% brinzolamide, are commonly administered alone or in combination.[24–29] In a large number of cases medical therapy alone is not enough to control the disease; in such cases surgery is indicated. Selective destruction of the ciliary body with laser (cyclophotoablation) transsclerally is intended to reduce aqueous humor production, whereas placement of gonioimplant shunts increase aqueous outflow.[32–37] In addition to specific glaucoma treatment,

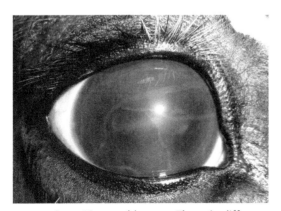

Fig. 4. Glaucomatous eye in a 19-year-old mare. There is diffuse corneal edema and numerous striae (Haab striae) caused by thinning of the Descemet membrane. The intraocular pressure at the time of diagnosis was 47 mm Hg. Note the abnormal pectinate ligament temporally.

therapy for the potential underlying ERU is essential. Chronically painful and blind glaucomatous eyes should undergo chemical ablation of the ciliary body by intravitreal injection of gentamicin or should be enucleated.[26]

THE LENS

The lens continues to grow throughout life by the sequential layering of new fibers around its nucleus.[38,39] Nuclear sclerosis, defined as the altered refractivity of the central lens observed in older animals caused by the compression of the central nucleus by enveloping fibers as part of the normal lens growth, has not been definitively described in horses.[12,38,39] However, cataracts, defined as any opacity or alteration in the optical homogeneity of the lens, are common in horses.[38] Cataracts were common findings in studies with geriatric horses and were present in up to 58.5% of horses more than 15 years of age.[3,40] When only those horses older than 30 years were considered, the prevalence of cataracts increased to 97%.[5]

The lens is rich in proteins called crystallines, which ensure its transparency.[38] Lens epithelial cells lose their organelles as they differentiate into fibers and with them their biosynthetic capacity. Therefore, lens fibers have a limited capacity to restore crystallines that may become damaged during the aging process.[41] Under normal conditions, the lens experiences years of exposure to factors such as ultraviolet light and chemical insult that are well known to destabilize proteins.[41] In addition, there is a loss of the redox balance of the major antioxidant system of the lens fibers. Once these crystallines are denatured, they condense into aggregates that induce light scatter and cause the white appearance of the lens in horses with cataracts.[41]

Typically, early senile cataracts appear as microvesiculation in the posterior suture lines. In older animals this progresses to more dense condensation around the posterior suture, together with perinuclear and cortical (anterior and posterior) cataracts.[12,38] Complete and occasionally hypermature cataracts can occur in some cases, with animals experiencing more significant visual compromise[12] (**Fig. 5**). Senile cataracts are usually bilateral but not necessarily symmetric.[38]

Although the use of antiinflammatories and antioxidants has been examined, the only treatment of cataracts is surgical removal of the lens.[38] Phacoemulsification is the technique of choice for lens removal in horses, with or without implantation of

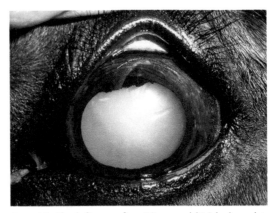

Fig. 5. Complete cataract in the left eye of an 18-year-old Irish draught mare. The lens was removed by phacoemulsification. Fourteen months after surgery the eye remains comfortable and visual. A faint perinuclear cataract was also present in the right eye in this mare.

an acrylic intraocular lens. However, surgery is typically reserved for those horses with a significant visual impairment.[42] Although the success rate for vision in the immediate postoperative period seems to be good, a recent study suggested that only 26.3% of horses remained visual 2 years after surgery.[43] However, this study considered horses lost to follow-up as nonvisual and therefore the long-term success rate may be higher. Another recent study found age not to be significantly associated with poorer outcomes following phacoemulsification, although horses older than 15 years had a lower visual outcome.[44] Intraocular inflammation is a potent cause of cataracts and therefore cataracts are a common consequence of ERU.[38] Horses with preoperative uveitis are significantly less likely to remain visual following phacoemulsification.[44]

THE VITREOUS

The vitreous occupies a great part of the ocular volume and has several important functions, including metabolic support and oxygenation, removal of the metabolic waste, and light transmission to the retina.[12,40] The vitreous is a clear, gel-like substance with a network of collagen fibrils that extend throughout the gel.[41] With aging, likely because of alteration or degradation of this collagen fiber network, there is a tendency for the gel to collapse; the vitreous attachments to the retina weaken and the space is filled with liquefied vitreous (termed syneresis).[16,41] In horses, true age-related liquefaction only happens in extreme old age; however, progressive dilution of the gel throughout life may give the impression of liquefaction from a fairly early age.[12] Two different studies in the United Kingdom found vitreous degeneration to be the most common ocular abnormality in geriatric horses, with a prevalence of 46% and 66% respectively.[3,40] Vitreous degeneration shows as clouding or discoloration of the vitreous gel with membranous or cellular debris that appears suspended within the vitreous body, sometimes termed floaters or muscae volantes.[12,45] In addition, inflammatory debris, often as a result of ERU, can contribute to vitreous opacity.[40]

Two other conditions of the vitreous seem to be more common in older horses. Asteroid hyalosis is a rare finding and manifests as white or refractive lipoid deposits within the vitreous gel structure, approximately 1 to 2 mm in size. These asteroid bodies remain suspended in the vitreous body but on occasions they move when the globe moves.[10,12,45] Synchysis scintillans or cholesterosis bulbi is also a rare condition, showing as multiple, highly refractile, golden particles formed by cholesterol crystals that flutter upward and then float back down with eye motion.[10,12,45]

THE RETINA

Several changes have been observed in the retinas of humans with aging. There is thickening of the internal limiting membrane and a decrease in the neural elements of the retina. The retinal pigment epithelium (RPE) may migrate into the sensory retina. The RPE may atrophy in areas surrounded by RPE hypertrophy and hyperplasia, thought to be as a result of insufficiency of the choroidal vasculature. There is also a gradual, age-related loss of rods.[16] Two significant changes have been observed in equine retinas of older horses compared with young horses. Large vacuoles, caused by bullous elevation of the epithelial cell layer, were detected at the level of the pars ceca retinae. The second change, observed in almost half of the retinas studied, was degeneration of the pars optica retinae with complete loss of the normal structure, affecting the first 0.5 mm of the retina from the border of the ora serrata.[46]

Senile retinopathy is the most common retinal condition found in older horses. Studies have shown a prevalence of between 33% and 42% in the general geriatric population; however, this prevalence increased to 73% when only horses older than 30 years were considered, suggesting a progressive nature.[3,5,40] In addition, the median age of horses affected bilaterally is significantly higher than the age of animals with unilateral lesions.[3] Senile retinopathy affects the retinal pigmented epithelium and photoreceptor layer and appears as irregular linear hyperpigmentation surrounded by hypopigmented areas, affecting typically the nontapetal fundus, although the tapetal fundus can also be involved[10,45,47,48] (**Fig. 6**). The pathogenesis of senile retinopathy is not fully understood but possible causes include oxidative damage or choroidal vasculature disease.[40] There is some debate as to whether senile retinopathy causes visual deficits or not. Some investigators think that this alteration is of no clinical significance, whereas others report problems with vision in the affected animals, particularly in poor lighting conditions.[12,47]

Inactive chorioretinitis lesions typically present as focal depigmented areas (so-called bullet-hole lesions) or as more extensive areas in the peripapillar region (butterfly lesions).[10,45,47,49] These lesions can be frequently found in young animals, but because they represent chorioretinal scars from previously active lesions is it likely that they present more commonly as horses get older. On some occasions they can cause visual deficits, but most often they represent an incidental finding.

Nonneoplastic masses of the optic nerve head also seems to be more common in older horses. Proliferative optic neuropathy appears as a white or pink lobulated mass at the edge of the optic nerve (**Fig. 7**). It is normally an incidental finding, although it may affect vision if it is big enough to obstruct the optic nerve head or central retina or when it results in continued movement (causing shying behavior).[10,45,47,48]

Exudative optic neuritis presents as sudden-onset bilateral blindness in horses more than 15 years of age.[10,47] On fundoscopic examination a lot of material can be seen extending from the surface of the optic nerve head towards the vitreous, with or without focal hemorrhages. If the optic disc is visible, it will appear swollen and edematous.

NEOPLASIA

Squamous cell carcinoma is the most common tumor of the eye and ocular adnexa in horses and there is an increased prevalence with age.[50] Risk factors include increased exposure to ultraviolet light and periocular hypopigmentation, although

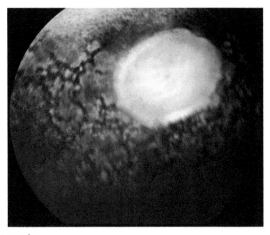

Fig. 6. Senile retinopathy.

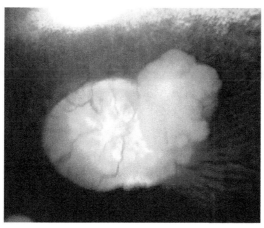

Fig. 7. Proliferative optic neuropathy in the right eye of a 15-year-old mare. This mare presented for examination for an unrelated condition. The owner reported no visual deficits and this was considered an incidental finding.

draught horse breeds with darkly pigmented periocular structures also show a higher incidence of the condition. In addition, geldings are 5 times more likely to develop ocular squamous cell carcinoma than stallions and twice more likely than mares.[50,51] The 2 most common locations are the third eyelid and the limbal conjunctiva[12] (Fig. 8) but any epithelial structure can be affected. Treatment of these tumors is challenging and frequently involves surgical excision followed by adjunctive therapy, including radiation, chemotherapy, and/or cryotherapy.[52] Recurrence following treatment is common.[10]

Melanoma is a common tumor in mature grey-coated or white-coated horses,[12,53,54] although it can affect horses with any coat color, and frequently affects the eyelids or other periocular structures. In contrast, most cases of intraocular melanoma tend to occur in younger horses between 5 and 10 years of age.[55] Early surgical removal of solitary early-stage melanomas affecting the eyelid is the recommended treatment[53,54] (Fig. 9). Other treatment options, with variable success rates reported, include intratumoral chemotherapy, immunotherapy, and cimetidine administration[53,54,56]

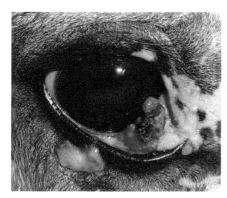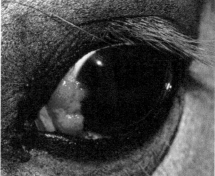

Fig. 8. Squamous cell carcinomas affecting the third eyelid of a 15-year-old Appaloosa gelding (*left*) and the nasal corneolimbal margin of a 17-year-old Haflinger mare (*right*).

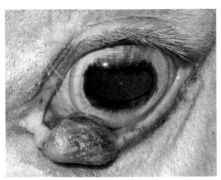 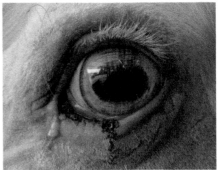

Fig. 9. Melanoma affecting the lower eyelid of a 16-year-old mare before (*left*) and after (*right*) surgical resection.

DISTURBANCES OF VISION

Objectively assessing vision in horses remains a challenge. Horses with significant ocular disease frequently show no behavioral changes that indicate visual compromise,[57] especially if the vision loss has developed over a long period of time.[2,57] This finding is particularly important in geriatric animals; these horses are usually managed in such a way, being kept in familiar surroundings and with a regular routine, that owners may miss early cues to visual impairment. The prevalence of owner-reported visual deficits in geriatric horses varies between 3.9% and 8% according to several studies,[2,4,40] but this number increased to 19% if only horses older than 30 years were considered.[5] Of these horses with owner-reported visual problems, veterinary examination showed that approximately half had a reduced pupillary light reflex and half had an absent or reduced menace response. Note that 1 of these studies showed that, despite the owners' concerns about the visual capacity of their horses, 50% were still used for ridden exercise, raising some important safety considerations.[2] In addition to the concerns for human safety, there are considerable animal welfare implications. Horses are naturally grazing animals that are hunted by predators and rely on vision as their primary sense. Blind horses, or those with significantly reduced vision, can show a high level of fear and anxiety; they can become unpredictable and require cautious handling by experienced caretakers.[58]

SUMMARY

Ocular abnormalities are a common finding in aged horses. Although these seldom cause overt visual deficits detected by their owners, they can be a source of chronic or acute discomfort so early detection, and treatment when available, is essential. Some of these abnormalities are specific to old horses, whereas others are a result of ongoing disorder or inflammation that started earlier in life but that becomes more evident when the damage sustained to the eye is advanced. If vision is significantly affected, consideration of human safety and animal welfare is paramount.

REFERENCES

1. Brosnahan MM, Paradis MR. Demographic and clinical characteristics of geriatric horses: 467 cases (1989-1999). J Am Vet Med Assoc 2003;223(1):93–8.

2. Ireland JL, Clegg PD, McGowan CM, et al. Comparison of owner-reported health problems with veterinary assessment of geriatric horses in the United Kingdom. Equine Vet J 2012;44(1):94–100.

3. Ireland JL, Clegg PD, McGowan CM, et al. Disease prevalence in geriatric horses in the United Kingdom: veterinary clinical assessment of 200 cases. Equine Vet J 2012;44(1):101–6.

4. Ireland JL, Clegg PD, McGowan CM, et al. A cross-sectional study of geriatric horses in the United Kingdom. Part 2: health care and disease. Equine Vet J 2011;43(1):37–44.

5. Ireland JL, McGowan CM, Clegg PD, et al. A survey of health care and disease in geriatric horses aged 30 years or older. Vet J 2012;192(1):57–64.

6. McGowan TW, Pinchbeck G, Phillips CJC, et al. A survey of aged horses in Queensland, Australia. Part 2: clinical signs and owners' perceptions of health and welfare. Aust Vet J 2010;88(12):465–71.

7. Michau TM, Schwabenton B, Davidson MG, et al. Superficial, nonhealing corneal ulcers in horses: 23 cases (1989-2003). Vet Ophthalmol 2003;6(4):291–7.

8. Gipson IK. Age-related changes and diseases of the ocular surface and cornea. Invest Ophthalmol Vis Sci 2013;54(14):48–53.

9. Crispin SM. Tear-deficient and evaporative dry eye syndromes of the horse. Vet Ophthalmol 2000;3(2–3):87–92.

10. Cutler TJ. Ophthalmic findings in the geriatric horse. Vet Clin North Am Equine Pract 2002;18(3):545–74.

11. Miller C, Utter ML, Beech J. Evaluation of the effects of age and pituitary pars intermedia dysfunction on corneal sensitivity in horses. Am J Vet Res 2013; 74(7):1030–5.

12. Chandler KJ, Matthews AG. Eye disease in geriatric horses. In: Bertone J, editor. Equine geriatric medicine and surgery. 1st edition. St Louis (MO): Saunders Elsevier; 2006. p. 173–8.

13. Brunott A, Boeve MH, Velden MA. Grid keratotomy as a treatment for superficial nonhealing corneal ulcers in 10 horses. Vet Ophthalmol 2007;10(3):162–7.

14. Lassaline-Utter M, Cutler TJ, Michau TM, et al. Treatment of nonhealing corneal ulcers in 60 horses with diamond burr debridement (2010-2013). Vet Ophthalmol 2014;17:76–81.

15. Hempstead JE, Clode AB, Borst LB, et al. Histopathological features of equine superficial, nonhealing, corneal ulcers. Vet Ophthalmol 2014;17:46–52.

16. Grossniklaus HE, Nickerson JM, Edelhauser HF, et al. Anatomic alterations in aging and age-related diseases of the eye. Invest Ophthalmol Vis Sci 2013; 54(14):ORSF23–7.

17. Rebhun WC. Corneal dystrophies and degenerations in horses. Compend Contin Educ Vet 1992;14(7):945–50.

18. Gilger BC, Deeg C. Equine recurrent uveitis. In: Gilger BC, editor. Equine ophthalmology. 2nd edition. St Louis (MO): Elsevier Saunders; 2011. p. 317–49.

19. Szemes PA, Gerhards H. Study on the prevalence of equine recurrent uveitis in the Cologne-Bonn area. Prakt Tierarzt 2000;81(5):408–20.

20. Dwyer AE, Crockett RS, Kalsow CM. Association of leptospiral seroreactivity and breed with uveitis and blindness in horses - 372 cases (1986-1993). J Am Vet Med Assoc 1995;207(10):1327–31.

21. Malalana F, Stylianides A, McGowan C. Equine recurrent uveitis: human and equine perspectives. Vet J 2015;206:22–9.

22. Gilger BC, Wilkie DA, Clode AB, et al. Long-term outcome after implantation of a suprachoroidal cyclosporine drug delivery device in horses with recurrent uveitis. Vet Ophthalmol 2010;13(5):294–300.
23. Curto EM, Gemensky-Metzler AJ, Chandler HL, et al. Equine glaucoma: a histopathologic retrospective study (1999-2012). Vet Ophthalmol 2014;17(5): 334–42.
24. Annear MJ, Gemensky-Metzler AJ, Wilkie DA. Uveitic glaucoma in the horse. Equine Vet Educ 2012;24(2):97–105.
25. Ollivier F, Monclin S. Equine glaucomas. Equine Vet Educ 2010;22(6):299–305.
26. Ollivier FJ, Sanchez RF, Monclin SJ. Equine glaucomas: a review. Equine Vet Educ 2009;21(5):232–5.
27. Thomasy SM, Lassaline M. Equine glaucoma: where are we now? Equine Vet Educ 2015;27(8):420–9.
28. Wilkie DA. Equine glaucoma: state of the art. Equine Vet J Suppl 2010;(37):62–8.
29. Wilkie DA, Gilger BC. Equine glaucoma. Vet Clin North Am Equine Pract 2004; 20(2):381–91.
30. Holve DL. Effect of sedation with detomidine on intraocular pressure with and without topical anesthesia in clinically normal horses. J Am Vet Med Assoc 2012;240(3):308–11.
31. Marzok MA, El-Khodery SA, Oheida AH. Effect of intravenous administration of romifidine on intraocular pressure in clinically normal horses. Vet Ophthalmol 2014;17:149–53.
32. Miller TL, Willis AM, Wilkie DA, et al. Description of ciliary body anatomy and identification of sites for transscleral cyclophotocoagulation in the equine eye. Vet Ophthalmol 2001;4(3):183–90.
33. Annear MJ, Wilkie DA, Gemensky-Metzler AJ. Semiconductor diode laser transscleral cyclophotocoagulation for the treatment of glaucoma in horses: a retrospective study of 42 eyes. Vet Ophthalmol 2010;13(3):204–9.
34. Cavens VJK, Gemensky-Metzler AJ, Wilkie DA, et al. The long-term effects of semiconductor diode laser transscleral cyclophotocoagulation on the normal equine eye and intraocular pressure. Vet Ophthalmol 2012;15(6):369–75.
35. Gemensky-Metzler AJ, Wilkie DA, Weisbrode SE, et al. The location of sites and effect of semiconductor diode trans-scleral cyclophotocoagulation on the buphthalmic equine globe. Vet Ophthalmol 2014;17:107–16.
36. Townsend WM, Langohr IM, Mouney MC, et al. Feasibility of aqueous shunts for reduction of intraocular pressure in horses. Equine Vet J 2014;46(2): 239–43.
37. Wilson R, Dees DD, Wagner L, et al. Use of a Baerveldt gonioimplant for secondary glaucoma in a horse. Equine Vet Educ 2015;27(7):346–51.
38. Matthews AG. The lens and cataracts. Vet Clin North Am Equine Pract 2004; 20(2):393–415.
39. Matthews AG. Lens opacities in the horse: a clinical classification. Vet Ophthalmol 2000;3(2–3):65–71.
40. Chandler KJ, Billson FM, Mellor DJ. Ophthalmic lesions in 83 geriatric horses and ponies. Vet Rec 2003;153(11):319–22.
41. Petrash JM. Aging and age-related diseases of the ocular lens and vitreous body. Invest Ophthalmol Vis Sci 2013;54(14):54–9.
42. Townsend WM. Cataracts: clinical presentations, diagnosis and management. Equine Vet Educ 2015. http://dx.doi.org/10.1111/eve.12388.
43. Brooks DE, Plummer CE, Carastro SM, et al. Visual outcomes of phacoemulsification cataract surgery in horses: 1990-2013. Vet Ophthalmol 2014;17:117–28.

44. Edelmann ML, McMullen R Jr, Stoppini R, et al. Retrospective evaluation of phacoemulsification and aspiration in 41 horses (46 eyes): visual outcomes vs. age, intraocular lens, and uveitis status. Vet Ophthalmol 2014;17:160–7.
45. Nell B, Walde I. Posterior segment diseases. Equine Vet J Suppl 2010;(37):69–79.
46. Ehrenhofer MCA, Deeg CA, Reese S, et al. Normal structure and age-related changes of the equine retina. Vet Ophthalmol 2002;5(1):39–47.
47. Cutler TJ, Brooks DE, Andrew SE, et al. Disease of the equine posterior segment. Vet Ophthalmol 2000;3(2–3):73–82.
48. Matthews AG, Crispin SM, Parker J. The equine fundus. III: pathological variants. Equine Vet J Suppl 1990;(10):55–61.
49. Mathes RL, Burdette EL, Moore PA, et al. Concurrent clinical intraocular findings in horses with depigmented punctate chorioretinal foci. Vet Ophthalmol 2012; 15(2):81–5.
50. Dugan SJ, Curtis CR, Roberts SM, et al. Epidemiologic study of ocular adnexal squamous cell carcinoma in horses. J Am Vet Med Assoc 1991;198(2):251–6.
51. Malalana F, Knottenbelt D, McKane S. Mitomycin C, with or without surgery, for the treatment of ocular squamous cell carcinoma in horses. Vet Rec 2010; 167(10):373–6.
52. Surjan Y, Donaldson D, Ostwald P, et al. A review of current treatment options in the treatment of ocular and/or periocular squamous cell carcinoma in horses: is there a definitive "best" practice? J Equine Vet Sci 2014;34(9):1037–50.
53. Moore JS, Shaw C, Shaw E, et al. Melanoma in horses: current perspectives. Equine Vet Educ 2013;25(3):144–51.
54. Phillips JC, Lembcke LM. Equine melanocytic tumors. Vet Clin North Am Equine Pract 2013;29(3):673.
55. Hollingsworth SR. Diseases of the uvea. In: Gilger BC, editor. Equine ophthalmology. 2nd edition. Louis (MO): Elsevier Saunders; 2011. p. 267–81.
56. Laus FC, Cerquetella M, Paggi E, et al. Evaluation of cimetidine as a therapy for dermal melanomatosis in grey horse. Isr J Vet Med 2010;65(2):48–52.
57. Matthews AG. Eye examination as part of the equine prepurchase examination. Equine Vet Educ 2015. http://dx.doi.org/10.1111/eve.12425.
58. Dwyer AE. Practical management of blind horses. In: Gilger BC, editor. Equine ophthalmology. 2nd edition. St Louis (MO): Elsevier Saunders; 2011. p. 470–81.

Integumentary Disorders Including Cutaneous Neoplasia in Older Horses

Derek C. Knottenbelt, OBE, BVM&S, DVM&S, MRCVS

KEYWORDS

- Skin • Tumor • Geriatric • Dermatology • Melanoma • Carcinoma • Pemphigus
- Sarcoidosis

KEY POINTS

- Older horses have few well-defined skin disorders apart from hypertrichosis/hirsutism associated with pituitary pars intermedia dysfunction and some neoplastic conditions.
- Several well-recognized diseases are known to show progressive deterioration in older horses; for example, insect-bite hypersensitivity.
- Tumors affecting older horses include melanoma and squamous cell carcinoma.
- Secondary skin disorders arising as a result of poor management or degrees of immuno-compromise can present in older horses.

INTRODUCTION

The skin of the horse is a highly visible and accessible organ that can reflect the overall health status of the horse or be affected by primary or secondary diseases. In a disease survey of 200 geriatric horses ($\geq$15 years of age) 71% had a dermatologic abnormality and 22% displayed hirsutism or abnormal shedding. Although the dermatologic abnormalities were not specifically identified/diagnosed, many were secondary bacterial, fungal, and parasitic infections (possibly related to degrees of immunocompromise) or neoplastic.[1] A recent pathologic study showed that in 4.2% the causes of death or euthanasia of animals more than 15 years of age were attributable to skin disease, including sarcoid, melanoma, lymphoma, and squamous cell carcinoma, and most of these were cutaneous.[2]

Several immune-mediated and autoimmune conditions affect older horses in particular but few of these are the preserve of older horses. Pemphigus foliaceus is probably the commonest autoimmune condition of horses and although the disease can affect horses of all ages, including the very young, it is generally regarded as being more serious from a prognostic perspective in older horses. Sarcoidosis (generalized

Equine Internal Medicine, University of Glasgow, Weipers Equine Centre Bearsden Road, Glasgow G611QH, Scotland
E-mail address: knotty@liv.ac.uk

Vet Clin Equine 32 (2016) 263–281
http://dx.doi.org/10.1016/j.cveq.2016.04.005
0749-0739/16/$ – see front matter © 2016 Elsevier Inc. All rights reserved.

granulomatous disease) is an immune-mediated generalized disease that often has prominent cutaneous signs and again this is probably more common in older horses. Management failures, often deriving from neglect and poor body condition, may result in immune compromise and consequent opportunistic primary skin infections and infestations, including viral, bacterial, fungal, and parasitic skin disease that would not normally affect the mature horse. Horses that develop unusual or opportunistic infections of the skin should probably be explored clinically for underlying immune-compromising disease.

Skin disease can result in significant morbidity and mortality in geriatric horses. Early detection of the more serious disorders of the skin could be instrumental in reducing the welfare implications of the conditions and improving the life span of affected horses. When examining an older horse for skin disease it is important to remember the basic division of the potential differential diagnoses. The broad categories of disease affecting older horses are shown in **Table 1**. Few skin conditions are the preserve of older horses but some are more associated with advancing age. Conditions that specifically affect the skin of older horses and donkeys include:

- Benign/natural graying and diffuse hair loss
- Pituitary pars intermedia dysfunction (PPID)

Table 1
Disease groups and the common primary and secondary skin disorders that particularly affect older horses

	Group	Primary	Secondary
Noninfectious disease	Genetic	Loss of pigment/graying Mane and tail dystrophy	—
	Immune mediated	Alopecia areata Insect bite Hypersensitivity Pemphigus Sarcoidosis	Paraneoplastic pemphigus Paraneoplastic pruritus
	Endocrine	Pituitary pars intermedia dysfunction Thyroid dysfunction (hypoplasia)	Bacterial, fungal, parasitic infections are common
	Toxic	—	Hepatocutaneous syndrome
	Idiopathic	Proliferative/verrucose pastern dermatitis	—
Infectious disease	Virus	Papilloma	Papilloma
	Bacteria	Pastern dermatitis	Staphylococcal pyogranuloma and furunculosis
	Fungus	—	Dermatophytosis
	Parasitic	*Chorioptes equi*	Dermatophilosis
Neoplastic disease	Ectodermal tumors	Squamous cell carcinoma Melanoma	—
	Mesenchymal tumors	Sarcoid Mast cell tumor	—
	Blood cell tumors	Lymphoma Plasma cell myeloma	—

- Melanoma
- Squamous cell carcinoma

These disorders may occur in younger animals and even PPID has been diagnosed with some regularity in mature horses under the accepted 15-year-old lower age limit for geriatric status. Other conditions have a higher incidence in older horses (≥15 years of age) than in younger ones or are often more significant/serious in older horses, and these are listed in **Box 1**.

The diagnostic protocol for evaluation of a dermatologic case in general is broadly and specifically the same as for any case; a full history and a full-body-systems examination needs to be undertaken before a specific and more detailed dermatologic examination. The dermatologic examination usually focusses on the main presenting complaint. There are primary skin diseases that are limited to the skin and others that have a systemic implication. Similarly, there are systemic diseases that have

---

Box 1
Primary and secondary conditions that are more common or severe in geriatric horses

Primary conditions:

- Mane and tail dystrophy
- Alopecia areata
- Pigmentary changes including natural graying/fading syndromes, spotted leukotrichia, and vitiligo
- Insect-bite hypersensitivity
- Pemphigus foliaceus
- Sarcoidosis
- Verrucose pastern dermatitis
- Melanoma
- Squamous cell carcinoma
- Cutaneous lymphoma
- Mast cell tumor
- Sarcoid
- PPID

Secondary conditions:

- Hepatic-derived photosensitization
- Hepatocutaneous syndrome
- Viral papilloma (immune compromise)
- Bacterial dermatitis (staphylococcal pyogranuloma/hoof canker); immunocompromise/ management failures
- Fungal dermatitis (dermatophytosis/fungal granuloma): immunocompromise/management failures
- Parasitic infestation (*Chorioptes equi/Sarcoptes scabiei*); immunocompromise/management failures
- Paraneoplastic pemphigus
- Paraneoplastic pruritus

cutaneous manifestations and some of these are serious. Often the skin signs are the earliest recognizable evidence of any disorder, particularly in geriatric horses because subtle signs are often overlooked or attributed to old age and natural tissue degradation. This situation is further complicated by the limited ways in which the skin can respond to insult; different diseases may have similar clinical appearances. For example, occult sarcoid, dermatophytosis, and alopecia areata can look similar but the implications, treatment options, and prognoses are very different. Typically, there is strong tendency to use intuitive supposition in dealing with skin disease but the tendency to say "I have seen something like this before so it must be the same disease" should be avoided and a thorough examination performed in every case. The direct visibility of most conditions in horses with skin disease almost forces clinicians into making snap diagnoses but many skin conditions in older horses are secondary to more serious internal disease. Good examples of this include opportunistic viral, bacterial, fungal, or parasitic infections that follow in cases of PPID.

In equine dermatology it is usually possible to make a tentative diagnosis from a careful history and an exhaustive clinical assessment, not only of the skin but of the whole horse, so these two fundamental aspects are critical and especially so in older horses, in which the underlying disorders can be more subtle. The commonest mistakes that are made center on the perhaps understandable diversion to the most obvious clinical sign without undertaking a proper critical appraisal of the whole animal.

It is important to identify every clinical sign and try to categorize the skin lesions into one of 6 syndrome classes, although an older horse can have several of these coexisting. These are:

1. Pruritus
2. Alopecia and hair density alteration
3. Pigmentary changes
4. Dry dermatoses (scaling and flaking)
5. Eczematous or moist dermatoses (weeping and seeping)
6. Nodular skin disease (neoplastic/inflammatory/other)

Time spent in clinical assessment and the collection of appropriate diagnostic samples is never wasted; it is better to perform a full investigation and get the diagnosis completely right and then focus the treatment accordingly, even when there are multiple conditions that are coexisting. A good example of this would be provided by an older horse that is presented with pruritus, alopecia, scaling, and peripheral edema. Each of these could be caused by individual comorbidity but they could all derive from a single internal tumor that produces more than 1 paraneoplastic sign. Similarly, an older horse that is presented with pruritus identified as being caused by parasites could be immunocompromised as a result of PPID. Treating the parasites is important, but it is equally important to understand the cause for any abnormal or unusual clinical event. An old gelding presented for a preputial discharge may have a primary sheath infection but more likely there is a primary cause for secondary infection, such as a squamous cell carcinoma, or it might be immunocompromised (or both). Dermatologists need to be exceptional internists as well.

Because most skin disease is directly visible and usually accessible, it should be possible to perform any further tests that may be indicated as being helpful with a specific intention of ruling in or ruling out defined differential diagnoses. However, the collection of appropriate samples should be performed with careful thought about what is likely to provide the best diagnostic information and what is both sensible and economical. The concept of collecting every sample possible because one is bound to come up with the diagnosis is both professionally poor and often unhelpful or overtly misleading.

PRIMARY CONGENITAL/HEREDITARY DISEASE OF OLDER HORSES
Fading Appaloosa Syndrome

Summary
This condition is really a progressive disorder of pigmentation: the natural patterning and color distribution becomes less definite and the coat becomes generally paler overall. There is no treatment and no clinical implication. It is not an acquired disorder of pigmentation so there is no increased tendency to actinic dermatitis or carcinoma that is related to this condition.

Clinical features

- Progressive loss of cutaneous and hair pigmentation to the point at which the horse may be almost unrecognizable
- The characteristic dark patches and spots may fade completely

Main differential diagnoses

- Natural graying

Diagnostic confirmation

- The condition is otherwise asymptomatic and is characteristic of the breed

Management

- No management is effective and none is required

Prognosis

- There is no treatment required or possible
- Owners should be advised that it is likely to be slowly progressive but many cases stabilize in their early teen years

Mane and Tail Dystrophy

Summary
This obvious condition affects Appaloosa horses in particular and is characterized by progressive, and often profound, hair loss/thinning of the mane and tail in particular.

Characteristically the condition has no implication for the general body coat but similar hair loss can be associated with the non–age-related disorder alopecia areata. The condition is distinctive and recognized as being a normal event in certain lines of Appaloosa horses. However, from a histologic perspective there is a suggestion that it might represent and unusual form of alopecia areata.[3] The otherwise asymptomatic condition can be mistaken for several other states but the overall clinical presentation is pathognomonic, at least in Appaloosa horses. There is no suggestion that affected horses are more or less liable to secondary skin disease as result of mane and tail dystrophy.

Clinical features

- Progressive loss of tail and mane hairs without any evidence of pruritus or other skin-related signs
- Variable extent but usually marked changes

Main differential diagnoses

- Alopecia areata

Diagnostic confirmation

- Biopsy is usually unhelpful

Management

- There is no treatment of this condition and owners should be advised accordingly

Prognosis

- It is best viewed as a cosmetic disorder
- Affected horses should probably not breed but, given the prevalence of this disease in the Appaloosa population in particular, it is almost inconceivable that such an approach would be either tolerated or achievable

PRIMARY IMMUNOLOGIC DISORDERS OF OLDER HORSES
Alopecia Areata

Summary
Although this condition is not restricted to older horses it is commoner in horses more than 10 to 12 years of age. The condition is probably immune mediated but is an almost asymptomatic disorder of the hair follicle. There is a reported seasonal variation with more obvious signs in spring and summer. Appaloosa and quarter-horse breeds are possibly more affected.[4]

Clinical features

- Limited areas (usually roughly circular, at least to start with) or more extensive diffuse hair loss without any other clinical sign.
- The mane and tail can also be affected.
- There is no apparent effect on the hoof capsule of affected horses.

Main differential diagnoses

- Dermatophytosis
- Occult sarcoid

Diagnostic confirmation

- Biopsy
  ○ Prominent lymphocytic infiltration around the hair bulb in the early stages.
  ○ Once the condition has established there is almost no histologic evidence of the underlying condition.

Management

- There is no treatment of the condition and, although it is widely regarded as an immune-mediated disorder, there is no value in corticosteroids or immunosuppressive drugs.

Prognosis

- There are some cases that seem to resolve to some extent over time but most remain with focal, discrete, or wider areas of profound alopecia or hair thinning.

Insect Bite Hypersensitivity

Summary

Insect-bite hypersensitivity (also known as sweet itch) is a common disorder. Onset is usually between 3 and 8 years of age but with advancing years the condition becomes increasingly severe so that by the time horses reach their geriatric age the skin can be seriously damaged. This very characteristic seasonal pruritic disorder is associated with profound I and type III hypersensitivity reactions. There are genetic aspects to this disease, with a higher prevalence in the Icelandic pony, the Shire, and the Welsh mountain pony, but almost all breeds can be affected. This condition is usually but not exclusively caused by the *Culicoides* insect group. The condition is not treatable but is usually manageable by avoidance of exposure to the appropriate insects.

Clinical features

- Exposure-related pruritus: this can be extreme or milder and can affect localized areas of the skin surface. Affected horses show dramatic pruritus when exposed to the *Culicoides* midges. The itch usually subsides if the horse is brought in or is otherwise protected from insect attack.
- Affected horses may scratch at different areas of the body that correspond with the biting habits of the specific species of *Culicoides* to which they are sensitive.

Main differential diagnoses

- Swarm attack form insects such as flies and mosquitos; insect bites/stings
- Parasitic infestations including *Chorioptes equi*, *Sarcoptes scabiei*, and lice
- *Oxyuris equi* infection (perineal pruritus)
- Paraneoplastic pruritus
- Multisystemic eosinophilic epitheliotropic disease

Diagnostic confirmation

- The history of progressive seasonal and environment-related pruritus is almost pathognomonic but it is important to remember comorbidity issues as horses get older.
- Intradermal skin testing is possible and is much more meaningful when the local species of *Culicoides* can be used as the antigen. This method is far more reliable than serum immunoglobulin E tests, which are notoriously unreliable and should probably be avoided at the present time.

Management

- Avoidance of contact with the relevant insect/*Culicoides* is the best strategy by far; insect repellants and fly sheets, rugs, hoods and so forth are effective in many cases.
- Allergen-specific immunotherapy used as a desensitization program can be effective in the long term.
- Topical oral high-dose nicotinamide and a variety of herbal remedies such as garlic can be useful in a few cases; however, most horses do not respond to these measures.
- Note that strategies that solely prevent the horse from itching are probably not acceptable because there are serious welfare issues in that approach.

Prognosis
- The prognosis is guarded because cases can be severe under certain circumstances and the welfare issues from self-trauma and/or insufficient management can be significant.

Pemphigus Complex

Pemphigus foliaceus

Summary This is autoimmune disorder that affects horses of all ages but the more serious forms occur in older individuals. The trigger for the disorder is seldom identifiable but viral infection and other diseases may be involved. In older horses the paraneoplastic form of the disease is possibly one of the most serious types of pemphigus.

Clinical features
- Focal or more diffuse, localized, or extensive skin exfoliation and hair loss. The resulting scale can be severe or very mild in a few cases.
- Oral ulceration can be encountered; there may be some changes in the eyelid margins as well.
- The skin may feel warm to the touch and can have a boarded feel. There is usually no pain or pruritus associated with these signs when they are not complicated by secondary infection or by concurrent morbidity such as neoplastic disease.
- Weight loss and limb edema are common.

Main differential diagnoses
- The only important noninfectious differential diagnosis is sarcoidosis/generalized granulomatous disorder. It can be difficult to differentiate the two on clinical grounds alone.
- Dermatophytosis and the generalized forms of dermatophilosis can be broadly similar but are recognizable for their specific contagion and the circumstances under which they develop.

Diagnostic confirmation
- Skin biopsy is definitive in most cases but it is important to remember that up to 8 or 10 biopsy specimens should be obtained and that no washing or wiping of the skin should be undertaken before the biopsy because this almost always results in the loss of the diagnostic acanthocytes in the scale and crust.
- Biopsy also serves to differentiate the main alternative diagnoses very clearly.

Management
- Immunosuppression is the only treatment of any consequence. Usually this is based on the use of immunosuppressive doses of corticosteroids and in particular prednisolone.
  - A dose of oral prednisolone starting at 2 mg/kg every 24 hours in the mornings only is usually adequate to bring the condition under control. Thereafter the dose can be adjusted downward progressively until a minimum effective alternate-day dose is achieved. This is often around the 1 mg/kg dose and again should be administered every alternate day in the morning only.
  - Dexamethasone can also be used either by injection (this is not the preferred route) or orally. The dose is usually accepted at 0.2 mg/kg mornings only. Again the objective is to try to reduce the dose progressively until such time as a minimum effective alternate daily dose is achieved.

  ○ Azathioprine at 2 mg/kg loading dose orally followed by 2 mg/kg on alternate days can be a useful way of reducing the amount of corticosteroid reliance. Azathioprine is not usually effective on its own.
  ○ Gold salt injection can be very effective but there are difficulties with the unwanted side effects of this approach. The injections are made once monthly and a dose of 1 mg/kg is usually advised. Effectiveness can be variable.

Prognosis

- Long-term treatment is essential; there is seldom any possibility of remission without medication even though some cases do have periods of time when they seem to be much better. The difficulty with reducing the medication is that once exacerbation occurs following cessation of medication the prognosis is significantly reduced.
- The overall prognosis for older horses that develop pemphigus foliaceus is poor for several reasons. The reliance on corticosteroids in older animals is potentially dangerous and there can be secondary effects, including the iatrogenic induction of insulin resistance and consequent laminitis. In addition, many of these horses have underlying comorbidity, including PPID and possibly neoplasia.

Sarcoidosis

Summary

Sarcoidosis is the term given to a generalized granulomatous disorder in which there are cutaneous manifestations.[5,6] The condition is rarely diagnosed but may be more prevalent than is appreciated because many of the signs are attributable to other conditions as well. Older horses are commonly affected but some young ones can acquire the condition.

This is an immune-mediated generalized granulomatous disease that affects multiple organs and tissues, including the skin; usually the limbs are affected but some cases have generalized signs.

Clinical features

- Two main forms of the disease are recognized:
  ○ Cutaneous disease (localized or generalized)
    ▪ Localized or generalized thinning of the hair coat, exfoliation with prominent scale formation
    ▪ Weight loss and reduced performance
  ○ Systemic disease with or without nodule formation

Main differential diagnoses

- Pemphigus foliaceus
- Occult sarcoid
- Dermatophytosis
- Dermatophilosis

Diagnostic confirmation

- Skin biopsy is highly suggestive with prominent multinucleated giant cell formations in the affected skin.[6]

Management

- It is tempting to use corticosteroids but little beneficial effect is usually achieved.[6]

Prognosis

- The prognosis for all forms of this disease is always very guarded.
- The more extensive cutaneous and systemic forms of the disease carry a much worse prognosis and when nodules are present the outlook is even worse. However, there are many cases of affected animals surviving for an extended length of time and even in the long term when the condition affects limited areas of the skin only. There is the possibility that this is a different form of the disease so it is hard to make the judgment as to whether the outlook is always as bad as it is reported to be.

Coronary Band Dystrophy

Summary

Coronary band dystrophy is a chronic long-standing proliferative condition affecting the coronary band of 1 or more feet. The condition may affect limited areas of the coronary band and is more common in heavier horses and in older horses of all breeds. The condition has an insidious onset and most cases involve all 4 coronary bands and the ergots and chestnuts.

Clinical features

- Proliferation of the superficial layers of the coronary band (and if appropriate the chestnuts and ergots) is a cardinal feature of this disease. Ulceration over short or larger areas is common.
- Hoof wall quality deteriorates dramatically over the full course of the disease and does not seem to resolve with or without any treatment. Horizontal and vertical wall cracks are common. The periople is usually severely affected and the hoof wall becomes crumbly and grossly abnormal. Hoof nails and adhesives are not usually strong enough to retain the shoe effectively. Cracks and break-back are common and these may result in significant lameness and secondary infection of the sensitive components of the hoof wall.

Main differential diagnoses

- Pemphigus foliaceus
- Systemic lupus erythematosus–like syndrome

Diagnostic confirmation

- The histologic appearance of this condition is well recognized by pathologists but there are variations in the interpretation of coronary band biopsies. Biopsy from at least 6 sites on at least 2 of the affected limbs is necessary. It is usually best to obtain the biopsy from the quarters or heels to avoid the risk of coronary band injury resulting in hoof wall cracks

Management

- Management is restricted to maintaining hoof wall quality by dietary supplementation with biotin, methionine, and essential omega-3 oils, although their effectiveness is debated.
- Retinoid gel application to the coronary band may help in the short term and regular treatment may help to maintain some degree of hoof wall normality.
- Corticosteroids and other immunosuppressive drugs have little effect.

Prognosis

- The prognosis for affected horses is very guarded. Most cases eventually succumb to various hoof wall problems and, because the condition is best regarded as untreatable and chronic, all care and support has to be viewed as palliative. Nevertheless, some cases can survive for an extended length of time. Few have ever been reported to resolve or to improve sufficiently to allow the withdrawal of any supportive treatment and management.

PRIMARY ENDOCRINE DISORDERS OF THE SKIN OF OLDER HORSES
Pituitary Pars Intermedia Dysfunction (Equine Cushing Disease)

Summary

PPID is a very common, and perhaps inevitable, central nervous disorder of older horses. PPID was the most common specific diagnosis, based on the postmortem presence of hyperplasia or adenoma, and was the reason for euthanasia in 47.7% of 65 equids with PPID.[2] Coexisting conditions in equids with PPID that were identified in this study but were not considered the basis for euthanasia included skin and other neoplasms, skin and other infections, lameness, and chronic airway diseases.

Clinical features

- Hypertrichosis is a cardinal and well-recognized clinical feature of PPID and is often the most striking clinical sign. This sign may be accompanied by sweating and secondary skin infections, including dermatophilosis, dermatophytosis, or external parasites.
- On histology, horses affected by PPID have a predominance of hair follicles in a persistent anagen phase (growth) associated with a marked reduction in telogen phase follicles.[7] Horses treated with pergolide showed both improved shedding and proportions of anagen and telogen phase follicles that were not different from those of control horses.[7]

Main differential diagnoses

- Although this condition is widely regarded as the only pathologic condition that causes hypertrichosis in horses, a few other related causes involving pituitary disorder have also been reported to result in this sign, including secondary lymphoma.
- Primary bacterial, fungal, or parasitic skin infections.

Diagnostic confirmation

- The diagnosis of PPID is based on a panel of clinical signs, and basal, dynamic, and biochemical parameters.[8,9]

Management

- Management of the skin signs is a fundamental requirement for the welfare of the horse. Close, regular clipping and early detection of parasitic and bacterial/fungal infections are essential. Clipping also reduces the sweating aspect of the disease. Secondary signs such as pruritus, verrucose and eczematous changes, and scaling dermatosis can be incidental findings from comorbidity of primary disease.
- The general signs of the condition can usually be managed with other nursing care (parasite control, dental and farrier support) and long-term oral use of pergolide.

Prognosis
The overall prognosis for PPID remains guarded. Because it is a progressive but manageable disorder the outlook usually depends heavily on the quality of care provided.

PRIMARY NEOPLASTIC DISORDERS OF THE SKIN OF OLDER HORSES
Melanoma

Summary
Melanoma is a tumor that arises from naturally occurring melanocytes, which are the pigment-producing cells in the skin and other parts of the body. Melanomas occur in all mammals but are the second most common skin tumor encountered in horses; they comprise between 3.8% and 15% of all skin tumors. No clear predilection for gender or breed has been established but, although they can be encountered in other colors of horse, a marked predisposition has been extensively reported in gray horses. More than 80% of gray horses, some cremello, and a few nongray horses can be affected by various extents of tumor development.

Melanomas can be classified individually into several distinct types and subtypes based on their clinical and pathologic behavior and histologic features.[10]

- Benign-appearing collections of melanocytes located in the superficial dermis or dermoepidermal junction are classified as melanocytoma (melanocytic nevi).
- Tumors located within deep dermal locations composed of well-differentiated melanocytes that show dense cytoplasmic pigmentation and minimal malignant criteria are classified as dermal melanoma.
  - Dermal melanomas are further subdivided clinically into tumors composed of a few discrete masses or nodules and a more disseminated variant with multiple, frequently confluent, tumors (dermal melanomatosis).

Anaplastic Malignant Melanoma

Summary
Overall, more than 90% of melanotic tumors are benign at early initial presentation but more than 60% to 70% usually progress to more overt malignant behavior if left untreated.[11] At present there are no meaningful data on the potential quantitative histologic indicators of malignancy, such as mitotic index, cellular Ki-67 expression, nuclear atypia, or the extent of cell differentiation; many of these aspects are used in canine and human melanoma description. Differentiation between benign and malignant tumors is usually based on the physical appearance (presence or loss of pigmentation), local growth pattern (localized defined or invasive growth), and the presence/absence of systemic involvement.

Clinical features
A variety of well-recognized features are common.

- Melanocytic tumors are generally heavily pigmented but areas of depigmentation can be identified within many tumors; these represent less differentiated cell populations. Amelanotic or poorly pigmented tumors occur in both gray and nongray horses.
- Tumors in affected horses are often located in the perineal region, under the tail, within the prepuce, and particularly on the preputial reflection and internal lamina, within the lips and eyelid margins. Any skin site can be affected.
- Tumors can be localized in the deeper dermal tissues or may involve more superficial dermis and epidermal tissue.

- Tumors that involve superficial tissues often ulcerate through the epidermis as they progressively enlarge.
- Progressive tumor enlargement can also result in central portions becoming necrotic as they outgrow their blood supply. A tarry black and bloodstained discharge is a common outcome of ulceration.
- Internal lesions are common, with most being identified clinically in the parotid region (salivary gland and lymph nodes), guttural pouches (usually lateral walls), and in any major internal organs. Almost any clinical sign in a gray horse could be attributable to melanoma.
- Disseminated (metastatic) forms are rare but important.

Main differential diagnoses

- Nodular sarcoid
- Mast cell tumor
- Cutaneous and deep lymphoma
- Collagen granuloma

Diagnostic confirmation

The diagnosis of melanoma in equine patients is usually reliably made from the physical appearance of the lesions and the signalment (older/mature gray horses). Lesions that lack pigment or that occur in nongray horses usually rely on biopsy examination. Biopsy provides a definitive diagnosis simply from a direct smear (even a fine-needle aspirate).

- Histologic examination of biopsy samples also provides information on potential malignancy.

Management

Treatment options for horses with melanocytic tumors can be divided into local and systemic therapies (**Fig. 1**).

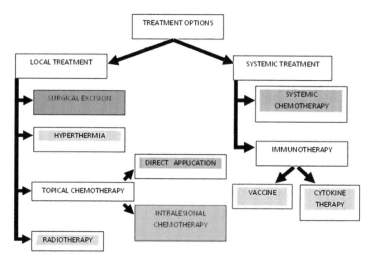

Fig. 1. The treatment choices for management of melanoma in horses. Options with green boxes have defined clinical evidence of efficacy. Pink boxes have evidence of some efficacy in some circumstances. Blue boxes indicate a lack of proven efficacy.

- Local therapy, including surgery, radiation, hyperthermia, and intralesional therapeutics, is usually used to treat isolated, defined, or uncomplicated tumors. Within this category it is possible to combine different therapies to achieve better overall outcomes.
- Surgical resection is generally considered the mainstay of therapy, but may not always be feasible. Surgical excision of all accessible and defined tumors is advisable at an early stage to preclude the subsequent transformation to malignancy or further risk of micrometastasis. Solitary or benign dermal melanomas are the most likely candidates for surgical resection. Surgery can also be used for more advanced tumors but typically involves tumor debulking and can be variably successful.
- Options for intralesional chemotherapy with cisplatin have been described and can be effective.[12] Cisplatin or carboplatin have been used with variable results. Usually these chemicals are delivered by intralesional injection of a slow-release form of the drug in sesame oil emulsion or as biodegradable beads.
- Systemic chemotherapy using oral cimetidine was reported to in one study to result in a dramatic improvement but no further studies have shown a similar benefit and it is now considered that this approach cannot be justified.[13] Nevertheless, there are anecdotal reports of some regression of some tumors in some horses.
- Radiation therapy has limited applicability and a poor response rate even when sophisticated radiotherapy methods are used. Radiation can be delivered by local interstitial brachytherapy using iridium[192] or by teletherapy. The former is rarely available and is best restricted to deep inaccessible tumors such as those in the soft tissues of the head and neck.
- Immunotherapy is the ultimate target for the treatment of this disorder. Clinicopathologic observations have suggested that equine melanoma in all its forms should be amenable to immunologic manipulation.[14] An early trial with an autochthonous vaccine reported dramatic responses but no further such outcomes have been reported since then. Options have been developed that specifically target functional enzymes or cytokines formed by the tumor. A xenogenic DNA vaccine encoding human tyrosinase (HuTyr), currently used to treat canine melanoma (Oncept, Merial), generates a tyrosinase-specific antitumor response. Although the vaccine is intended for use in dogs, in which it has been shown to improve survival, it has been shown to have significant effects in some equine cases.[15] In comparison, the equine tyrosinase sequence shares 90% homology with the human sequence; based on this, cross reactivity of HuTyr DNA vaccine in the horse is expected. The safety and activity of this vaccine has been evaluated in normal horses,[16] and this seems to be a major prospect for the future management of equine melanoma.

Prognosis

- Most melanoma lesions are slow growing and individual tumors have limited (but sometimes serious) space-occupying effects. For example, lesions in the cerebrum, brain stem, and spinal cord have profound effects. However, in most cases it is the confluent and malignant skin forms that create the biggest threat to the life of the horse.
- Most horses die with the disease rather than because of it.

Squamous Cell Carcinoma

Summary

Squamous cell carcinoma (SCC) is more prevalent in the older horse population, in which it can affect the skin at various sites such as the penis, prepuce, vulvar and perineal skin, the mouth, and the eyelids. Most commonly the affected cutaneous skin is nonpigmented. The most common sites for SCC to develop in older horses are the skin of the mouth and both male and female external genitalia. Penile and preputial SCC mainly affects older horses and most studies report an average age of 17 to 20 years.[17,18]

Carcinoma development has been attributed to the presence of bovine papilloma viruses but the relationship between the two conditions has not been definitively established. The virus can be found on normal sin and in particular on areas of inflamed or ulcerated skin in other conditions as well. The same relationship has been suggested for other forms of cutaneous and mucosal carcinoma. There is a strong relationship with nonpigmented skin at all sites where the condition develops apart from the vulvar and perineal forms, in which pigmented skin can also be affected.

Although carcinoma lesions of the skin of the face, mouth, and eyelids are usually seen early in their development, the early stages of penile tumors often remain undiagnosed, possibly for years, because lesions on these regions are easily missed by all but the most observant of owners. Horses are often presented with severe lesions that present with sanguineous or purulent discharge and a fetid odor caused by secondary infection and tissue/tumor necrosis. Localized preputial edema and even abnormal urination (spraying, dribbling, and straining) can also be the earliest signs recognized by owners.

Examination of any suspected carcinoma requires a thorough examination, including the regional lymph nodes if possible. In the case of the penile forms, the inguinal lymph nodes are frequently involved and in oral and palpebral forms the pharyngeal and diffuse tonsillar glands may be affected. Penile examination invariably requires the use of sedation with acetylpromazine (0.04–0.1 mg/kg intravenously) to promote penile protrusion.

Clinical features

- Ranges from the earliest squamous dysplasia and squamous papilloma to the most serious, highly destructive fungating carcinoma.
- Carcinoma of the skin is a progressive condition and so the early signs can be misleadingly benign. Ulcerated or proliferating (papillomatous) lesions, particularly on nonpigmented skin or mucosae, should arouse suspicion of early carcinoma.
- The most obvious sign of penile or preputial carcinoma is usually a persistent, fetid, purulent preputial discharge. Blood-stained or dark brown preputial discharge is sometimes the first evidence of disease. Penile SCC usually presents as irregularities on the penile or preputial surface or nonhealing erosions with or without accompanied granulation tissue. In more advanced stages, the tumor often presents as a solid mass with a cauliflowerlike appearance, and may contain large necrotic areas. The glans penis and the urethral fossa are commonly affected. In many horses, penile SCC is accompanied by penile papillomata (which are usually considered to be precancerous lesions) and by large, confluent, pink to yellowish plaques that are referred to as penile intraepithelial neoplasia (PIN) lesions.
- Eyelid and conjunctival carcinoma are characterized by an almost pathognomonic type of purulent discharge even in the earliest stages of development. Either ulcerating and destructive lesions or proliferative lesions resembling papilloma are usually visually obvious.

- Almost all carcinoma lesions affecting the lips and mouth are highly destructive and have a characteristic foul smell.
- Paraneoplastic or secondary effects can be seen later in the course of disease.
- Metastatic tumors are not common in any form but can present with internal organ involvement.

Main differential diagnoses

- Traumatic lesions
- Papilloma
- Sarcoid
- Ulcerated (amelanotic) melanoma
- Basal cell carcinoma
- Lymphoma

Diagnostic confirmation

- Biopsy is definitive and important because it establishes the grade of the lesion. All stages of the development are well recognized by pathologists.

Management

- The options for treatment are usually dictated by the location and stage or grade of the tumor.
- Surgical removal with or without concurrent topical or intralesional chemotherapy is probably the most common treatment method but is only applicable to defined locations where the surgical procedure is feasible.[12,19] Vulvar, penile, and (lower) eyelid lesions are amenable to surgery in most cases with varying surgical procedures being required. Typically, surgery has to have the objective of total removal of all affected tissue with a safe margin of excision. Local lymph node removal is a wise measure if feasible.
- Cryosurgery (with or without local or intralesional chemotherapy) has to be considered in smaller localized lesions such as the squamous dysplasia or PIN lesions on the penis.
- Topical and intralesional chemotherapy have been used extensively with good reported success rates.[12] Topical 5% 5-fluorouracil has good effect on penile carcinoma.[20,21] Topical mitomycin-C has been found to be effective in the treatment of ocular forms of carcinoma but it is suggested that it has a better effect when the tumor is first surgically reduced.[22,23] This suggestion is surprising because surgical tumor reduction improves the outlook for all forms of treatment. The value of cisplatin (and probably carboplatin) in the treatment of carcinoma by intralesional injection (using slow-release oil emulsions or biodegradable beads) has been proved.[24–26]
- Electrochemotherapy using cisplatin or 5-fluorouracil can significantly improve the outcome of chemotherapy in sarcoid tumors and it is likely that this is also a useful method of treatment in carcinoma.[27]
- Radiotherapy is known to be highly effective in the treatment of all forms of carcinoma.[28,29] The options include local brachytherapy (usually using high-dose or low-dose iridium[192]) or plesiotherapy (usually using strontium[90] or ruthenium). The problem is the availability of either low-dose or high-dose iridium[192] sources and facilities to handle them. Teletherapy systems are highly effective but logistically even more problematic.

- The therapeutic approach taken by attending veterinarians must consider several short-term and long-term implications. However, it is always best to use the best available treatment as a first approach because failure results in a reduced prognosis both locally and for the patient.

Prognosis

- The prognosis depends heavily on the stage of the tumor and the duration of the condition. However, when carcinoma is detected early and treated appropriately, there can usually be the expectation of a successful outcome.
- Comorbidity (eg, with PPID or other immunocompromising states) results in a significant reduction in prognosis.
- Severe or functionally limiting tumor development carries a worse prognosis than tumors that develop slowly in convenient anatomic sites.
- Local lymph node involvement suggests malignancy and reduced outlook and definite metastatic spread carries a hopeless prognosis. It is important to differentiate inflammatory/responsive lymphadenopathy from metastatic spread and so local lymph node biopsy or submission of excised lymph nodes (if feasible) should always be performed.

SUMMARY

- When dealing with skin disease in older horses no potential diagnosis should be excluded and a full clinical work-up is always indicated. Primary and secondary skin disease is common in older horses when comorbidity and poor management combine.
- By far the commonest specific skin disorder of older horses is the hypertrichosis/hirsutism associated with PPID (Cushing disease). Because this disease results in significant long-term immunocompromise, opportunistic/secondary skin infections are common in older horses with PPID.
- There are several well-recognized skin immune-mediated disorders that become significantly worse with advancing age, such as insect-bite hypersensitivity.
- Skin tumors are probably more common in older horses; melanoma and carcinoma are the most prevalent skin tumors restricted to older horses. Other skin tumors are less commonly associated specifically with old age.

REFERENCES

1. Ireland JL, Clegg PD, McGowan CM, et al. Disease prevalence in geriatric horses in the United Kingdom: veterinary clinical assessment of 200 cases. Equine Vet J 2012;44:101–6.
2. Miller MA, Moore GE, Bertin FR, et al. What's new in old horses? Postmortem diagnoses in mature and aged equids. Vet Pathol 2016;53(2):390–8.
3. Von Tscharner C. Stannard's illustrated equine dermatology notes. Vet Dermatol 2000;11:161–205.
4. Hoolahan DE, White SD, Outerbridge CA, et al. Equine alopecia areata: a retrospective clinical descriptive study at the University of California, Davis (1980-2011). Vet Dermatol 2013;24:282-e264.
5. Sloet van Oldruitenborgh-Oosterbaan MM, Grinwis GC. Equine sarcoidosis. Vet Clin North Am Equine Pract 2013;29:615–27.
6. Sloet van Oldruitenborgh-Oosterbaan MM, Grinwis GC. Equine sarcoidosis: clinical signs, diagnosis, treatment and outcome of 22 cases. Vet Dermatol 2013;24:218–24.e48.

7. Innerå M, Petersen AD, Desjardins DR, et al. Comparison of hair follicle histology between horses with pituitary pars intermedia dysfunction and excessive hair growth and normal aged horses. Vet Dermatol 2013;24:212–7.

8. McGowan TW, Pinchbeck GP, McGowan CM. Prevalence, risk factors and clinical signs predictive for equine pituitary pars intermedia dysfunction in aged horses. Equine Vet J 2013;45:74–9.

9. McGowan TW, Pinchbeck GP, McGowan CM. Evaluation of basal plasma α-melanocyte-stimulating hormone and adrenocorticotrophic hormone concentrations for the diagnosis of pituitary pars intermedia dysfunction from a population of aged horses. Equine Vet J 2013;45:66–73.

10. Valentine BA. Equine melanocytic tumours: a retrospective study of 53 horses (1988 to 1991). J Vet Intern Med 1995;9:291–7.

11. Moore JD, Shaw S, Beuchner-Maxwell V, et al. Melanoma in horses: current perspectives. Equine Vet Educ 2013;25:144–51.

12. Théon AP, Wilson WD, Magdesian KG, et al. Long-term outcome associated with intratumoral chemotherapy with cisplatin for cutaneous tumors in equidae: 573 cases (1995-2004). J Am Vet Med Assoc 2007;230:1506–13.

13. Goetz TE, Ogilvie GK, Keegan KG, et al. Cimetidine for the treatment of melanoma in 3 horses. J Am Vet Med Assoc 1990;196:449–52.

14. Jeglum KA. Melanomas. In: Robinson NE, editor. Current therapy in equine medicine. Philadelphia: WB Saunders; 1997. p. 399–401.

15. Brazil TJ. Melanoma–where are we now and what does the future hold? Proc Br Equine Vet Assoc 2015;147.

16. Lembcke LM, Kania SS, Blackfors JT, et al. Development of immunogenic assays to measure response in horses vaccinated with xenogenic plasmid DNA encoding human tyrosinase. J Equine Vet Sci 2012;32:607–15.

17. van den Top JGB, Harkema L, Lange C, et al. Expression of p53, Ki67, EcPV2- and EcPV3 DNA, and viral genes in relation to metastasis and outcome in equine penile and preputial squamous cell carcinoma. Equine Vet J 2015;47:188–95.

18. Martens A. Tumors of the equine male urogenital tract. Proc Am Coll Vet Surg 2015;567–9.

19. Van den Top JGB, de Heer N, Klein WR, et al. Penile and preputial tumours in the horse: a retrospective study of 114 affected horses. Equine Vet J 2008;40:528–32.

20. Patterson S. Treatment of superficial ulcerative squamous cell carcinoma in three horses with topical 5-fluorouracil. Vet Rec 1997;141:626–8.

21. Fortier LA, MacHarg MA. Topical use of 5-fluorouracil for treatment of squamous cell carcinoma of the external genitalia of horses: 11 cases (1988-1992). J Am Vet Med Assoc 1994;205:1183–8.

22. Rayner SG, van Zyl N. The use of mitomycin C as an adjunctive treatment for equine ocular squamous cell carcinoma. Aust Vet J 2006;84:43–6.

23. Malalana F, Knottenbelt DC, McKane SA. Mitomycin C, with or without surgery, for the treatment of ocular squamous cell carcinoma in horses. Vet Rec 2010;167:373–6.

24. Hewes CA, Sullins KE. Use of cisplatin-containing biodegradable beads for treatment of cutaneous neoplasia in equidae: 59 cases (2000-2004). J Am Vet Med Assoc 2006;229:1617–22.

25. Théon AP, Pascoe JR, Carlson GP. Intratumoral chemotherapy with cisplatin in oily emulsion in horses. J Am Vet Med Assoc 1994;202:261–4.

26. Théon AP, Pascoe JR, Madigan JE. Comparison of intratumoral administration of cisplatin versus bleomycin for treatment of periocular squamous cell carcinoma in horses. Am J Vet Res 1997;58:431–3.
27. Tamzali Y, Borde L, Rols MP, et al. Successful treatment of equine sarcoids with cisplatin electrochemotherapy: a retrospective study of 48 cases. Equine Vet J 2012;44:214–20.
28. Théon AP. Radiation therapy in the horse. Vet Clin North Am Equine Pract 1998; 14:673–88.
29. Plummer CE, Smith S, Andrew SE, et al. Combined keratectomy, strontium-90 irradiation and permanent bulbar conjunctival grafts for corneolimbal squamous cell carcinomas in horses (1990-2002): 38 horses. Vet Ophthalmol 2007;10: 37–42.

Cardiac and Respiratory Disease in Aged Horses

Celia M. Marr, BVMS, MVM, PhD

KEYWORDS

- Respiratory • Cardiac • Recurrent airway obstruction • Thoracic neoplasia
- Valvular disease • Echocardiography • Electrocardiography

KEY POINTS

- Respiratory and cardiac disease are common in older horses.
- Advancing age is a specific risk factor for cardiac disease.
- Recurrent airway obstruction can lead to irreversible structural change and bronchiectasis and, with chronic hypoxia, right heart dysfunction and failure can develop.
- Valvular heart disease often affects the aortic and/or the mitral valve; it does not necessarily shorten life span, but can progress to congestive heart failure.
- Management of comorbidity is an essential element of the therapeutic approach to cardiac and respiratory disease in older equids.

 Video content accompanies this article at http://www.vetequine.theclinics.com.

AGE AS A RISK FACTOR FOR CARDIAC AND RESPIRATORY DISEASE IN HORSES

Respiratory disease is common in the geriatric horse: horse owners reported that 14% of 918 horses of aged 15 years or over coughed[1] and in a survey involving 67 horses of 30 years or over, owners reported 8% of their horses had respiratory problems, with this being the second most common reported problem after lameness.[2] In the same survey, 86% of the respiratory cases required at least 1 veterinary visit in the preceding year,[2] and in another survey of horse owners, 25% of 165 horses of 20 years or older were receiving medication of which around 1 in 5 was owing to lower airway disease.[3] Although there is slight agreement among owner and veterinary assessment of respiratory health status in older horses,[4] the assessments of prevalence of respiratory disease based on veterinary examination indicate higher prevalence than those based on owner questionnaires. Veterinarians frequently identified cough (7.5%), nasal discharge (17.5%), and abnormal respiratory sounds on rebreathing that were marked (14%) or moderate (18%) in a group of 200 horses of 15 years or older.[5]

Funding and Competing Interests: None to declare.
Rossdales Equine Hospital and Diagnostic Centre, Cotton End Road, Exning, Newmarket, Suffolk CB8 7NN, UK
E-mail address: celia.marr@rossdales.com

Horses with abnormal findings with rebreathing were older than those that did not, with median ages of 21 years and 18 years, respectively.[5] Respiratory diseases were also common in horses 20 years or older admitted to a veterinary teaching hospital and this was the third most common body system involved, after gastrointestinal and musculoskeletal problems.[6] Recurrent airway obstruction (RAO) was diagnosed in 6% of this patient group, 2% had laryngeal disease, and 2% pneumonia usually related to episodes of esophageal obstruction.[6]

Cardiac disease is also fairly common in the geriatric horse, but horse owners are less likely to recognize this in their geriatric horses. Only one of the owners of 200 horses that were 15 years or older reported that his or her horse had a cardiac murmur when in fact cardiac murmurs were detected in 20%.[4] In a study of the very old horse population, more than one-third had murmurs unrecognized by the owners.[2] The prevalence of murmurs of left-sided valvular regurgitation (LSVR) increases with age[7] and age and male sex are risk factors for aortic regurgitation (AR).[8] Compared with small ponies, there was a greater prevalence of LSVR in small, Thoroughbred-type horses.[7] Researchers have not consistently grouped age and use various forms of classification of cardiac murmurs when reporting findings, but in horses 15 or older to 23 years and 24 years or older, LSVR was found in 13.5% and 14.8%,[7] a study of horses of 15 years or older, documented cardiac murmurs in 20%[5] and another survey focusing on horses 30 years or older, reported murmurs consistent with AR in 19%, mitral regurgitation (MR) in 17% and tricuspid regurgitation was rare, with around 5% always occurring in horses with additional left-sided murmurs.[2] Irregularity of cardiac rhythm, consistent with atrial fibrillation (AF), was detected on auscultation in 2% of horses of 15 years or older[5] and greater than 4.4% of horses 30 years or older.[2] Age is not a specific risk factor for AF,[8] although MR is recognized as a predisposing condition for this arrhythmia in general[9] and MR increases the likelihood of recurrence of AF.[10] It is likely that the majority of elderly horses with AF have some degree of underlying structural heart disease and, therefore, treatment recommendations aiming to correct the arrhythmia that apply in athletes,[11] often with lone AF, do not translate to the geriatric patient group.

Although morbidity is high, cardiovascular and respiratory diseases are relatively rarely the cause of death in older horses, representing 4.6% and 4.2%; gastrointestinal disease (42%) and neoplasia (19%) were the most common causes of death in a recent survey of post mortem findings in 241 equids.[12] There was no difference in mortality of horses with and without murmurs of LSVR in a 4-year longitudinal study and owner-reported cause of death was related to the cardiovascular system in only 8%.[7]

SPECIFIC CONDITIONS
Recurrent Airway Obstruction

RAO is a multifactorial disorder, affecting horses from fairly early in life. The overall disease prevalence has been estimated to be around 14% in one UK study, although horses 15 years or older are much more likely to be affected, with an odds ratio of 18.3 (95% CI, 4.31–77.66) compared with horses younger than 5 years.[13] Residence in an urbanized environment, respiratory infection, and exposure to hay/straw early in life were additional risk factors.[13] RAO is characterized by hypersensitivity-mediated, neutrophilic airway inflammation and lower airway obstruction. It is recurrent in nature and clinical signs tend to be prompted by exposure to airborne organic dust.[14] Most veterinarians are only too familiar with the clinical signs, diagnosis, and management of RAO (**Fig. 2**A). Cough and nasal discharge are common, but the absence of these signs does not rule out neutrophilic airway inflammation.[15] Severely and chronically affected individuals may have hypertrophy of the abdominal muscles ("heaves line"), nasal flare, and wheezes and crackles.

Uncomplicated geriatric RAO cases are generally managed in the same way as cases in other age groups. Most veterinarians prefer to confirm the diagnosis on the basis of airway cytology and findings on tracheal endoscopy.[14] Histamine broncho-provocation can be used to confirm airway obstruction and, unlike neutrophil counts in bronchoalveolar lavage fluid, abnormal results can be expected in horses in remission as well as those with active clinical signs.[15,16] Plethysmography together with histamine challenge is usually used to identify airway reactivity. Aging does not seem to affect results.[17] Although less well-characterized, plethysmography can be used to document whether horses respond to bronchodilators. Delta flow is a measure of airway obstruction derived from respiratory inductive plethysmography with RAO.[17] In most horses with RAO, albuterol will be associated with an improvement in indicators flow-derived indexes.[18–21] Failure to improve delta flow by more than around 20%, measured 5 and 20 minutes after administration of 500 μg via metered dose inhaler suggests that there may be structural change in the airways and a poor prognosis is warranted (Nolen-Watson, personal communication, 2013). Conversely, with the severely affected older patient, the ability to document objectively that bronchodilation can be achieved can provide motivation and help owners to decide whether they want to introduce bronchodilator therapy.

Specific details of environmental management and therapy for RAO have been reviewed extensively elsewhere[14] and are beyond the scope of this paper. Corticosteroids are commonly used with favorable results. In the geriatric patient, comorbidity is common and it may be prudent to consider the possibility of pituitary pars intermedia dysfunction (PPID)[22] before embarking on corticosteroid therapy. In milder cases, environmental change alone or together with sodium chromoglycate given via metered dose inhaler (8–12 mg)[23] can be helpful, but in more severe RAO cases, it may not be possible to avoid using corticosteroids even in the presence of PPID. Although inhaled corticosteroids are an attractive option because they are less likely to have systemic effects, with severe RAO a course of systemic corticosteroids is often required before inhaled corticosteroid therapy can be initiated for long-term maintenance.[23] Clearly, the owner must be made aware of risks associated with this approach, but in some cases the benefits of corticosteroids in controlling inflammation associated with RAO may outweigh potential risks of laminitis in a patient, which may also have laminitis risk associated with PPID.

Bronchiectasis

Bronchiectasis is a pathologic process rather than a specific disease entity involving irreversible dilation of the bronchi or bronchiole that is associated with airway inflammation, destruction of the airway architecture, accumulation of mucus, and bacterial infection.[24] It is rare in horses, but older horses are at risk. Three horses have been reported in the equine veterinary literature, aged between 12, 15, and 17 years. Two of these horses had been first diagnosed with RAO, at least 4 and 7 years previously[24] and this is a condition that should be considered when horses with long-standing RAO deteriorate, become unresponsive to corticosteroid therapy, lose weight, or develop fever. Radiographs demonstrate distended bronchi, particularly in the caudal lung field (**Fig. 1**). Treatment is aimed at environmental dust control together with antiinflammatory therapy. Antimicrobials are indicated if secondary bacterial infection is present. The prognosis is guarded: 2 of the 3 horses that have been documented improved.

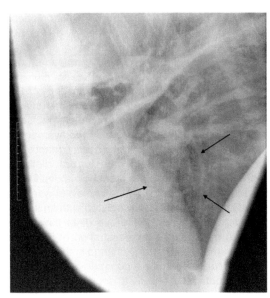

Fig. 1. A lateral thoracic radiograph demonstrating the caudoventral lung field from a 15 year-old New Forest Gelding with a long-standing history of recurrent airway obstruction that had developed recent lethargy and fever. Distended bronchi (*arrows*) indicate bronchiectasis.

Hypoxia and Right Heart Dysfunction

In response to hypoxia, pulmonary vasoconstriction and pulmonary hypertension can develop. These changes are reversible,[25] but with chronic hypoxia, ultimately right heart failure can ensue[26–28] and this process has been reported primarily as a sequel to long-standing RAO in elderly horses. If right heart failure is present, there are typically clinical signs such as jugular distension and pulsation, but the clinical presentation also generally includes severe respiratory compromise, reflecting the underlying cause. In horses in the reversible stages, pulmonary hypertension may be suspected based on echocardiographic signs, including increase in the pulmonary artery diameter relative to the diameter of the aortic root (**Fig. 2**B), increased right ventricular diameter, decreased left ventricular diameter, and paradoxic septal motion (**Fig. 2**C).[25] Aggressive treatment of the underlying respiratory problem, including intranasal oxygen therapy, can resolve the pulmonary hypertension (**Fig. 2**D). However, if the right heart fails, the prognosis is poor.

Pneumonia in the Older Horse

Pneumonia in the older horse can be related to aspiration,[6] but PPID is also an important predisposing cause: horses with PPID may be immunosuppressed and pneumonia is common in these cases.[22] It has been suggested that occult infections may occur with PPID because of the absence of a significant inflammatory response to pathogens[22] and, interestingly, the airway inflammation has been suggested as a possible contributing factor to the development of PPID because chronic inflammation and oxidative stress have been associated with neurodegeneration.[29] The pathogenic events and mechanisms linking pulmonary disease and PPID remain to be determined; nevertheless, such horses may not necessarily have obvious signs of respiratory disease and therefore a high index of suspicion is necessary and tracheal

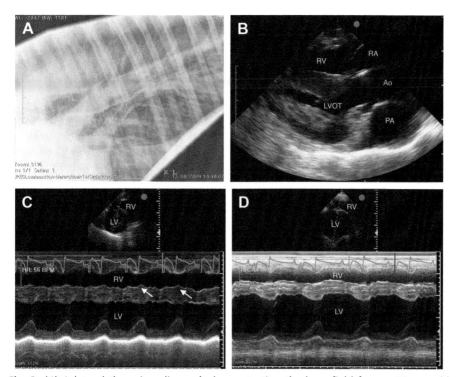

Fig. 2. (*A*) A lateral thoracic radiograph demonstrating the lung field from a 16-year-old pony mare with dyspnea, tachypnea, tachycardia, and jugular distension. The vasculature is prominent and there is a marked bronchointerstitial pattern consistent with recurrent airway obstruction. (*B*) A right parasternal long axis 2-dimensional echocardiogram of the left ventricular outflow tract (LVOT). The diameter of the pulmonary artery (PA) is large relative to the aorta (Ao), suggesting pulmonary hypertension. RA, right atrium; RV, right ventricle. (*C*) An M mode echocardiogram of the right (RV) and left ventricles (LV) with corresponding 2-dimensional image showing cursor placement. The RV diameter is large relative to the LV and paradoxic septal motion is present, such that the septum moves upwards toward the RV in systole (*arrows*). (*D*) Initially, the pony (*C*) was treated with intranasal oxygen for 48 hours and dexamethasone and ipratropium for 1 month. This M mode echocardiograph obtained at 30 days shows the paradoxic septal motion is no longer present and the RV is less dilated.

cytology. Thoracic radiographs and/or thoracic ultrasound examinations should be considered in horses with PPID that are debilitated with no localizing signs to avoid missing comorbidity. Therapy for pneumonia involves broad-spectrum antimicrobials, ideally guided by culture and antimicrobial sensitivity patterns. Therapy aimed at control of PPID if present will improve prognosis.

Aortic Valvular Regurgitation

In the middle-aged and geriatric horse, the aortic valve is the commonest site for degenerative valvular pathology,[30,31] which in turn can be associated with regurgitation. Nodular or, less commonly, generalized fibrous thickenings can affect any or all 3 valve cusps, but are seen most often on the left coronary cusp.[30–33] The murmur of AR is typically pan-, holo-, or early diastolic decrescendo with its point of maximal intensity over the aortic valve in the left fifth intercostal space and radiates variable distances ventrally toward the heart base. It is often musical or it can have a bizarre 'creaking' quality, which may be owing to vibrations of cardiac structures, such as the mitral valve and the ventricular septum, rather than turbulent blood flow itself.[34] Horses with severe AR are likely to have loud diastolic murmurs and often there are multiple heart murmurs if there is degenerative change in more than 1 valve.[35]

The quality of the arterial pulses is a very useful guide to severity of AR: as AR increases in severity, left ventricular volume overload develops and this is reflected as hyperkinetic pulse quality with a strong systolic component with rapid transition to low diastolic pressures owing to the retrograde flow of AR. It can also be useful to measure noninvasive arterial pressure, which provides a useful guide to severity and horses with severe AR are have diastolic arterial pressure of less than 50 mm Hg and a pulse pressure (ie, systolic – diastolic) of greater than 60 mm Hg compared with horses with mild AR.[35] As the AR progresses to insufficiency, increases in resting heart rate may also be observed.

In many horses, AR is well-tolerated and it is often an incidental finding in middle-aged and older horses and AR in isolation was not associated with congestive heart failure (CHF) in a study of risk factors for cardiac disease in an equine hospital population.[8] When advising on the significance of AR in the older horse, the clinician must consider the horse's activity and workload. In geriatric horses that are retired, further investigations may not be required; however, with older horses still in work, a more detailed appraisal of AR is warranted. In a recent American College of Veterinary Internal Medicine/European College of Equine Internal Medicine consensus statement, it was recommended that horses with severe AR should not be ridden or driven by a child, used as a lesson horse, or participate in a high-risk sport owing to a risk for sudden cardiac death and these comments may be applicable to a subset of geriatric patients.[11]

Echocardiography is the primary tool for investigation of equine valvular disease. The 2-dimensional and M mode echocardiographic features of AR have been described extensively.[33,36,37] With degenerative disease, there may be nodular or generalized thickening of the aortic valve (**Figs. 3**A and **4**A, B, Videos 1 and 2), valvular prolapse (see **Fig. 3**A, Video 1) and flail cusp. Dilatation of the aortic root (>8 cm), diastolic vibrations of the mitral valve (**Figs. 3**B and **4**C) and septum, and premature closure of the mitral valve (see **Fig. 3**B), are seen with moderate to severe AR but are not necessarily related to severity.[33] Color flow Doppler echocardiography can give a subjective impression of the severity of AR. Horses with AR had significantly larger and faster regurgitant jets found with spectral Doppler echocardiography if a cardiac murmur was present, suggesting that these parameters do reflect severity to some extent.[36] With large jets, flow moving toward the regurgitant orifice progressively increases in velocity, shown with color flow Doppler as bands of color and aliasing as it approaches the orifice. This is used in human cardiology to assess severity of valvular regurgitation and various parameters have been validated for this purpose. In horses, these methods have not been validated, but proximal flow convergence is generally only observed with moderate or severe AR (see **Figs. 3**C and **4**D; Videos 3 and 4). Critically, the degree of left volume overload is an important indicator of severity and is identified if the left ventricular diameter is increased, and the ventricle is hyperkinetic (Video 5). M mode echocardiography is the most precise method to measure left ventricular dimensions (**Fig. 3**D, E) but left ventricular volume overload can also be subjectively assessed with 2-dimensional echocardiography as typical the apex of the ventricle takes on a globoid shape (**Fig. 3**F, see Video 5). In horses with very advanced AR, the left ventricle may fail, leading to reduced septal and free wall movement.

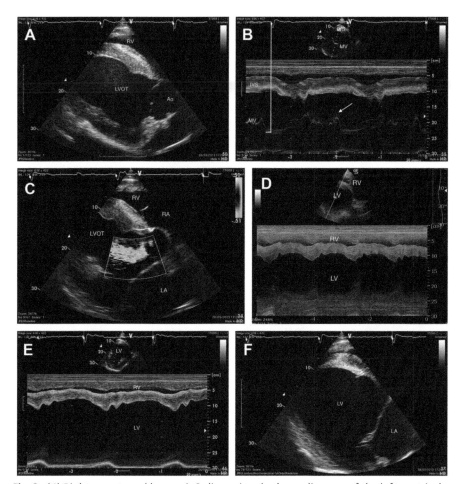

Fig. 3. (*A*) Right parasternal long axis 2-dimensional echocardiogram of the left ventricular outflow tract (LVOT) from a 20-year-old Thoroughbred stallion. The aortic valve is nodular and prolapses and the left ventricle is rounded (see Video 1 for corresponding images). Ao, aorta; RV, right ventricle. (*B*) An M mode echocardiograph of the mitral valve (MV) with a corresponding 2-dimensional image showing cursor placement demonstrated diastolic vibrations of the MV (*arrow*) and premature MV closure (indicated by lines from point of valve closure to Q wave). IVS, interventricular septum. (*C*) A slightly oblique, long axis 2-dimensional echocardiogram of the LVOT showing part of a large jet of aortic regurgitation (AR). Note the apical portions of this regurgitant jet extend beyond the sample area used in this image (see Video 3 for corresponding image). LA, left atrium; RA, right atrium. (*D, E*) M mode echocardiograms of the LV from a Thoroughbred stallion with AR. The images were obtained 5 years apart and show that there has been considerable increase in the diameter of the LV. At the time the second image was obtained (*E*), the horse was aged 20 years, his murmur had increased from grade 3 to grade 4 but the horse was not showing any external signs of cardiac dysfunction and the AR and left ventricular volume overload was not impacting on his quality of life and he was still able to breed. (*F*) A right parasternal long axis 2-dimensional echocardiogram which shows that the LV is dilated and very rounded at the apex in this 20-year-old stallion with AR (see Video 5 for corresponding images).

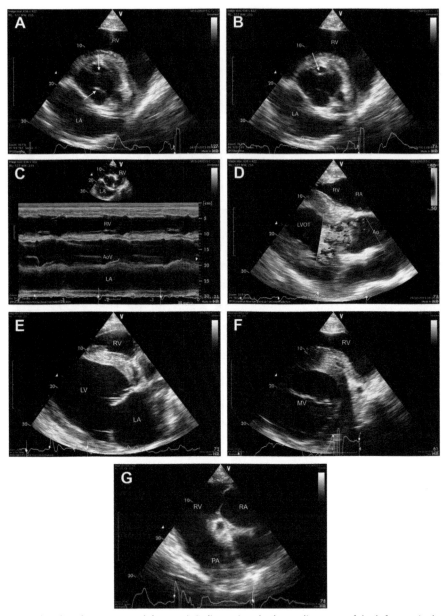

Fig. 4. (*A, B*) Right parasternal short-axis 2-dimensional echocardiograms of the left ventricular (LV) outflow tract from a 19-year-old Warmblood gelding. At different phases of the cardiac cycle (indicated by the red line on the electrocardiograph [ECG]), nodular changes (*arrows*) can be seen on the aortic valve cusps (see Video 2 for corresponding images). LA, left atrium; RV, right ventricle. (*C*) An M mode echocardiogram of the aortic valve (AoV) with a corresponding 2-dimensional image showing diastolic vibrations of the valve due to aortic regurgitation (AR). (*D*) Right parasternal long axis color flow Doppler echocardiogram of the left ventricular outflow tract (LVOT) showing marked proximal flow convergence and jet of AR (see Video 4 for corresponding image). Ao, aorta; RA, right atrium. (*E, F*) Right parasternal long (*E*) and short (*F*) axis 2-dimensional echocardiograms of the LA, LV, and RV from the same horse showing the horse also has generalized thickening of the mitral valve (MV), confirming degenerative changes in both mitral and aortic valves. Note the ECG shows atrial fibrillation. (*G*) A right parasternal inflow–outflow 2-dimensional echocardiogram showing that, in this horse with both aortic and mitral regurgitation, the pulmonary artery (PA) is dilated.

An apparent association between AR and ventricular dysrhythmias has been reported.[35,38] This seems to be independent of the severity of AR, although supraventricular premature depolarizations are more likely to be seen in horses with severe AR.[35] It has also be suggested that AR can lead to sudden cardiac death in horses with moderate to severe AR and can occur in isolation, without a history of poor performance or CHF.[11] Therefore, ambulatory and exercising electrocardiography should be included the diagnostic workup in cases of AR that are being used for riding purposes and horses with ventricular dysrhythmias are considered less safe for athletic use than their age-matched peers.[11] Owners of geriatric AR patients are often very willing to use heart rate monitors during exercise and this can give some level of assurance that the horse is not being asked to undertake excessive work. Various products are available that record the heart rate via devices embedded in girth attachments The geriatric horse owner can be encouraged to devise a personalized "standard exercise test" to record the heart rate over a specific distance and location where they regularly ask the horse to work at is hardest; for example, this might be cantering up a hill that they regularly visit. Veterinary advice should be sought if the resting heart rate consistently exceeds around 45 bpm, and typical heart rates at the trot are around 80 to 120 bpm, collected canter 120 to 150 bpm, fast canter 150 to 180 bpm, and maximal gallop 200 to 230 bpm. The advantage of performing this regularly at home is that trends over time can be identified, but veterinarians should be aware that they may not be able to differentiate very high heart rates and, of course, these devices record rate not rhythm.

Mitral Regurgitation

The mitral valve is the second commonest location for valvular pathology, most often related to degenerative valvular disease.[30,39] MR can arise secondary to dilation of the valve annulus,[39] for example, as a result of severe AR and degenerative change can affect more than one valve concurrently (**Fig. 4E–G**). MR is the commonest form of equine cardiac disease detected in referral centers and is the form of valvular regurgitation most likely to be associated with AF,[9] clinically significant ventricular arrhythmias, pulmonary regurgitation, and CHF.[8,40] Slowly progressive valvular disease is often well-tolerated until it becomes very severe, but chorda tendinea can rupture spontaneously or after inflammatory or degenerative disease leading to a rapid change in left heart hemodynamics that is much less well-tolerated.[40,41] MR can lead sudden death owing to pulmonary rupture, which is the result of pulmonary hypertension that ensues as MR leads first to increases in left atrial pressure and ultimately to increased pressure within the pulmonary circulation.[40]

The MR murmur is holosystolic or pansystolic, typically band shaped, is loudest over the left fifth intercostal space, and radiates variable distances caudodorsally. The grade of the murmur does not necessarily relate to the severity of the disease, and it may reflect the direction of the regurgitant jet, frequently being louder if the jet is orientated toward the chest wall, as opposed to the slightly more common caudodorsal direction. The degree of radiation of the murmur is an important guide to severity with more severe MR being audible over a wide area. Horses with more severe MR often have a loud third heart sound: the third heart sound relates to early ventricular filling and increases in its volume raise the suspicion that there may be increased left ventricular diastolic filling and left ventricular volume overload.[39]

Severe degenerative disease of the mitral valve typically produces generalized or nodular thickening on echocardiography[40,42] (see **Fig. 4E, F**). Portions of the chordae tendineae may flail into the left atrium with ruptured chorda tendinea.[40,43] These are usually found in left parasternal long axis images and a careful search across the entire valve plane is required as they may be seen in only 1 image. Flow mapping can underestimate the severity of MR, because it is difficult to align the ultrasound beam parallel to the direction of regurgitant flow (**Fig. 5**A, B, Video 6). Therefore, care must be taken if a small jet is detected in a horse with other signs of severe MR, such as left atrial enlargement or left ventricular volume overload. Echocardiographic signs consistent with left ventricular volume overload include increases in the left atrial diameter and enlargement of the left ventricle with rounding of its apex such that that the ventricle adopts a globular appearance (**Fig. 5**C, Video 7). The diameter of the pulmonary artery should be assessed as dilation is suggestive of pulmonary hypertension and may be a precursor to rupture, collapse and death[40] (see **Fig. 4**G). Myocardial disease may accompany mitral valve disease.[40] If this has led to severe dilatation, the prognosis is poor, particularly if the fractional shortening is decreased.

In many horses with MR owing to degenerative valvular disease, progression does occur, although it generally occurs slowly over months or years; thus, many geriatric cases are relatively untroubled by their heart disease. If the horse is still in vigorous work, the American College of Veterinary Internal Medicine/European College of Equine Internal Medicine guidelines on management of equine athletes with cardiovascular abnormalities may be relevant[11] and, as described, some owners will maintain horses with moderate or severe MR in light work using heart rate monitors. The

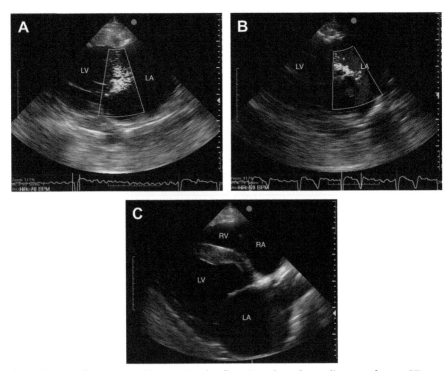

Fig. 5. (*A, B*) Left parasternal long axis color flow Doppler echocardiograms from a 27-year-old Thoroughbred gelding with mitral regurgitation. To delineate the full extent of the regurgitant flow the sample area has to be repositioned around the left atrium (LA; see Video 6 for corresponding images). Note the electrocardiograph shows atrial fibrillation. LV, left ventricle. (*C*) A right parasternal long axis 2-dimensional four chamber echocardiogram showing both the LV and LA are globular and subjectively enlarged (see Video 7 for corresponding images). RA, right atrium; RV, right ventricle.

presence of AF raises an additional concern because AF cases may have inappropriately high heart rates at exercise, ventricular dysrhythmias, and/or aberrant conduction.[44] To date, this has only been documented in horses with lone AF, but clinical experience suggests this can also occur in horses with underlying structural disease (**Fig. 6**). Therefore, if owners of geriatric horses with valvular disease and AF wish to continue to ride their horses, it may be prudent to perform several exercising electrocardiographic studies to evaluate the rhythm fully. Exercise-associated cardiac arrhythmias can be intermittent; again, this has not been evaluated specifically in the geriatric cardiac patient, but a small study in younger, healthy horses showed that performing more than 3 exercise tests, revealed a higher prevalence of postexercise arrhythmias, but arrhythmias during exercise were more repeatable. There was no difference in prevalence when treadmill and overground exercise tests were compared.[45] Thus, it is critical that owners of geriatric horses understand that significant arrhythmias can be intermittent and may not be detected during veterinary assessments.

Aortocardiac Fistula

With aortocardiac fistula (ACF) occurs a dissecting tract that develops from the aorta. The most common location is the right sinus of Valsalva, but occasionally it occurs in the noncoronary sinus. The tract can extend in various from the aorta to the right atrium, the right ventricle and/or the interventricular septum (**Fig. 7**, Videos 8 and 9). The precise cause is unknown; intact aneurysms may be present before the rupture[46] and the lesion may relate to congenital or acquired degeneration of the media of the aorta.[47,48] Some reports have associated the condition with chronic AR with aortic root dilation but, given the relatively high prevalence of AR, it is possible both these conditions could coexist without necessarily being related.[49] Although ACF can occur at any age, many affected animals are middle-aged or older and males seem to be more prone to this condition than females.[50]

ACF can present as sudden death, often during breeding or exercise; acute thoracic pain, which can be mistaken for abdominal pain; and CHF.[49–52] The murmur of ACF is a low-pitched and continuous with its point of maximal intensity over the right hemithorax. Ventricular tachycardia is common, most likely owing to disruption of the conducting tissue by a tract extending into the interventricular septum.[50] Some cases may have AF relating to atrial dilation (see **Fig. 7**, Videos 8 and 9). The prognosis is poor, although horses have been reported to survive the initial episode for periods of up to 2 years after diagnosis of this condition.[49,50,52,53] Horses with ACF should not be ridden because they are at risk of sudden death.[11]

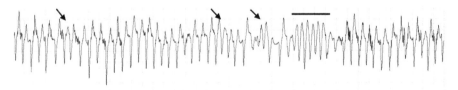

Fig. 6. An electrocardiograph obtained during lungeing exercise from a 16-year-old Irish draft/Thoroughbred gelding with severe mitral regurgitation and atrial fibrillation. The horse is trotting but the heart rate is inappropriately high, averaging around 200 bpm with some instantaneous rates of almost 300 bpm. Several wide ventricular complexes are present (some examples indicated with *arrows*) and there is a run of ventricular complexes with R-on-T (*under line*).

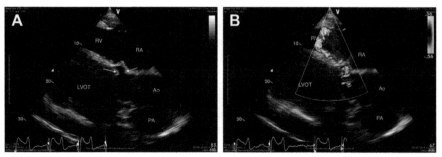

Fig. 7. (*A*) Right parasternal long axis echocardiogram of the left ventricular outflow tract (LVOT) from an 18-year-old polo pony gelding with an aortocardiac fistula (between *arrows*) tracking from the right sinus of Valsalva to the right ventricle (RV). The electrocardiograph (ECG) shows atrial fibrillation (see Video 8 for corresponding images). Ao, aorta; PA, pulmonary artery; RA, right atrium. (*B*) Right parasternal long axis color-flow Doppler echocardiogram of the LVOT from an 18-year-old polo pony gelding. An intracardiac shunt is visible tracking through an aortocardiac fistula from the right sinus of Valsalva to the RV. The ECG shows atrial fibrillation (see Video 9 for corresponding images).

Thoracic Neoplasia

Neoplasia is an important cause of death in the geriatric horse, accounting for almost 20% of deaths in 1 survey[12] in which squamous cell carcinoma, lymphoma, and melanoma were the most common malignant neoplasms and all have potential for thoracic involvement.[54,55] Advancing age increased the odds of diagnosis of all 3 of these tumors compared with sarcoids. However, examination of the relative proportions of tumor types diagnosed in horses in recent years shows that there has been an increase in other tumors, probably reflecting that there is now more veterinary and owner interest in undertaking investigations in older horses compared with previous decades.[56] The pulmonary granular cell tumor is the commonest form of primary lung tumor in horses (**Fig. 8**). A specific age effect has not been document, but most reports of this form of neoplasia have been in older horses.[57–59]

Clinical signs of thoracic neoplasia are often fairly nonspecific, but this should be suspected with weight loss, increased respiratory rate and effort, and intermittent

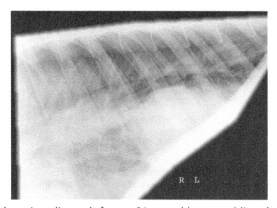

Fig. 8. A lateral thoracic radiograph from a 21-year-old pony gelding that presented with intermittent epistaxis. There is a soft tissue opacity within the left lung which is due to pulmonary granular cell tumor.

fever. With cranial thoracic masses, there may be jugular distension, epistaxis may be present with pulmonary neoplasia (see **Fig 8; Fig 9**), and cutaneous hyperthermia and localized sweating on 1 side of the head owing to sympathetic denervation at the cervicothoracic ganglion has been associated with melanoma. Thoracic ultrasonography is useful for identification of pleural effusion, cranial thoracic masses (**Fig. 10**), and lung lesions that extend to the periphery of the lung (**Fig. 11A**). Thoracic radiography may demonstrate pulmonary lesions (see **Figs. 8, 9** and **11A**). Ante mortem confirmation of diagnosis relies on cytologic or histologic examination of fluid or biopsied masses. There is 1 report of successful transendoscopic electrosurgery of a pulmonary granular cell tumour,[60] but for the majority of cases of thoracic neoplasia, therapy is not indicated or feasible and only palliative care is available.

SPECIFIC CONSIDERATIONS FOR THERAPY FOR GERIATRIC PATIENT WITH CARDIAC AND/OR RESPIRATORY DISEASE
Congestive Heart Failure

CHF should be suspected in horses presenting with ventral edema, often relating to the sheath and ventral abdomen, venous distension and jugular pulsation, poor arterial pulse quality and resting heart rates of 50 bpm or greater. Coughing is fairly rare in CHF, although it may be present with acute onset left heart failure; however, radiography may demonstrate interstitial edema in many horses with CHF. In geriatric horses, CHF usually relates to structural heart disease and because the most common form, degenerative valvular disease usually very slow progressive course, by the time signs of CHF are evident, the underlying pathology may have existed for many years. Nevertheless, management of CHF in the short and medium term can be effective. In the long term, it is rarely successful: 9 of 14 horses presenting in CHF were euthanized and the remainder died or were euthanized within 1 year.[26]

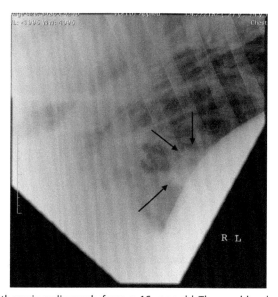

Fig. 9. A lateral thoracic radiograph from a 16-year-old Thoroughbred gelding that presented with intermittent epistaxis and subcutaneous swellings biopsied from which had been diagnosed as hemangiosarcoma. There is a soft tissue opacity visible just caudal to the heart (*arrows*).

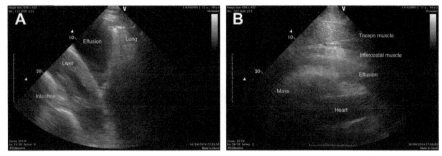

Fig. 10. (*A*) Thoracic ultrasonography demonstrates pleural effusion with atelectasis of the ventral portion of the lung in an 18-year-old Thoroughbred gelding with cranial mediastinal lymphoma. This diagnosis was confirmed ante mortem by cytologic examination of the pleural fluid. (*B*) In the same horse, ultrasound images of the cranial mediastinum obtained by imaging through the muscles caudal to the shoulder demonstrated effusion and a soft tissue mass cranial to the heart.

The general goals of therapy in CHF are to improve cardiac output and reduce congestion. The renin–angiotensin–aldosterone system, endothelin, and beta-adrenoceptors activation are all potential sites for pharmacologic intervention to improve cardiac output. The normal equine myocardium primarily expresses beta-1 adrenoreceptors but heart failure increases the expression of beta-2 adrenoceptors.[61] There is currently no species-specific evidence to support the use of beta-blocking agents in horses but sotalol, a nonselective beta-adrenergic receptor blocker that also has potassium channel blocking antiarrhythmic effects has become popular among equine cardiologists recently. Pharmacokinetic studies have yet to be published and therefore the appropriate dose is unknown but anecdotally, it is often used at around 2 to 3 mg/kg orally. Sweating is common for the first few days of treatment; sotalol can be proarrhythmic[62,63] and should be avoided in patients with renal disease.[64]

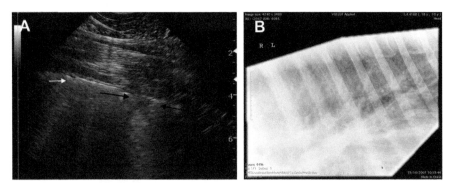

Fig. 11. (*A*) Thoracic ultrasonography demonstrates multifocal lesions at the periphery of the lung in a 20-year-old Hanoverian gelding with multicentric lymphoma and lymphoblastic leukemia. In this example, the black arrows indicated one of the larger lesions, of around 1 cm diameter and the white arrow indicate a comet tail, which was widespread throughout the lungs. (*B*) Thoracic radiographs from the same horse show a diffuse interstitial pattern throughout the lungs which is military in appearance. Post mortem examination confirmed obliteration of the normal lung parenchyma by a massive infiltration of dysplastic lymphocytes.

The angiotensin-converting enzyme inhibitor quinapril, given orally at a dose of 120 mg/horse per day, led to increased stroke volume and cardiac output and a reduction in the amount of valvular regurgitation, but no clinically significant changes in cardiac size after 8 weeks of therapy in horses with mitral insufficiency but no CHF. This corresponded with an owner-reported improvement in exercise tolerance.[65] Another angiotensin-converting enzyme inhibitor, enalapril, has poor oral bioavailability.[66,67] Recently, the pharmacokinetics for pimobenan have been reported for horses.[68] This drug is a calcium sensitizer and a selective inhibitor of phosphodiesterase III. The vasodilator effect decreases the resistance to blood flow, decreasing afterload that should, in turn, reduce the amount of MR. In healthy horses a dose of 0.25 mg/kg administered intragastrically had positive chronotropic and inotropic effects.[68]

Reducing congestion is generally tackled with diuretics and furosemide is the most widely used diuretic in horses. Furosemide is usually administered at 1 to 2 mg/kg 2 to 3 times per day intravenously or intramuscularly. In many horses it is effective orally; occasionally, however, beneficial effects abate when the route of administration is changed from intravenous to oral. Long-term administration may produce hyponatremia, hypokalemia, hypomagnesaemia, and metabolic alkalosis.[69] Therefore, periodic monitoring of serum electrolyte concentrations is advisable during furosemide therapy.

Comorbidity in the Geriatric Patient

Management of comorbidity is an important consideration when managing geriatric equines. There may be relatively little that can be done to specifically address pathologies such as degenerative valvular disease but attention to patient's additional health problems may have a dramatic and beneficial effect on the horse's overall quality of life. Multifocal musculoskeletal disease, dental problems, and concurrent cardiac and respiratory disease are frequently found together in the aged horse and it is important that the specialist clinician does not focus exclusively on cardiac or respiratory disease alone and overlook opportunities to review the horse's preventive health care program and to address those additional problems that can be managed effectively.

SUPPLEMENTARY DATA

Supplementary data related to this article can be found at http://dx.doi.org/10.1016/j.cveq.2016.04.006.

REFERENCES

1. Ireland JL, Clegg PD, McGowan CM, et al. A cross-sectional study of geriatric horses in the United Kingdom. Part 2: health care and disease. Equine Vet J 2011;43:37–44.
2. Ireland JL, McGowan CM, Clegg PD, et al. A survey of health care and disease in geriatric horses aged 30 years or older. Vet J (London, England: 1997) 2012;192: 57–64.
3. Brosnahan MM, Paradis MR. Assessment of clinical characteristics, management practices, and activities of geriatric horses. J Am Vet Med Assoc 2003;223:99–103.
4. Ireland JL, Clegg PD, McGowan CM, et al. Comparison of owner-reported health problems with veterinary assessment of geriatric horses in the United Kingdom. Equine Vet J 2012;44:94–100.
5. Ireland JL, Clegg PD, McGowan CM, et al. Disease prevalence in geriatric horses in the United Kingdom: veterinary clinical assessment of 200 cases. Equine Vet J 2012;44:101–6.

6. Brosnahan MM, Paradis MR. Demographic and clinical characteristics of geriatric horses: 467 cases (1989-1999). J Am Vet Med Assoc 2003;223:93–8.

7. Stevens KB, Marr CM, Horn JN, et al. Effect of left-sided valvular regurgitation on mortality and causes of death among a population of middle-aged and older horses. Vet Rec 2009;164:6–10.

8. Leroux AA, Detilleux J, Sandersen CF, et al. Prevalence and risk factors for cardiac diseases in a hospital-based population of 3,434 horses (1994-2011). J Vet Intern Med 2013;27:1563–70.

9. Reef VB, Levitan CW, Spencer PA. Factors affecting prognosis and conversion in equine atrial fibrillation. J Vet Intern Med 1988;2:1–6.

10. Decloedt A, Schwarzwald CC, De Clercq D, et al. Risk factors for recurrence of atrial fibrillation in horses after cardioversion to sinus rhythm. J Vet Intern Med 2015;29:946–53.

11. Reef VB, Bonagura J, Buhl R, et al. Recommendations for management of equine athletes with cardiovascular abnormalities. J Vet Intern Med 2014;28:749–61.

12. Miller MA, Moore GE, Bertin FR, et al. What's new in old horses? Postmortem diagnoses in mature and aged equids. Vet Pathol 2016;53(2):390–8.

13. Hotchkiss JW, Reid SWJ, Christley RM. A survey of horse owners in Great Britain regarding horses in the their care: part 2: risk factors for recurrent airway obstruction. Equine Vet J 2007;39:301–8.

14. Pirie RS. Recurrent airway obstruction: a review. Equine Vet J 2014;46:276–88.

15. Rettmer H, Hoffman AM, Lanz S, et al. Owner-reported coughing and nasal discharge are associated with clinical findings, arterial oxygen tension, mucus score and bronchoprovocation in horses with recurrent airway obstruction in a field setting. Equine Vet J 2015;47:291–5.

16. Vandenput S, Votion D, Duvivier DH, et al. Effect of a set stabled environmental control on pulmonary function and airway reactivity of COPD affected horses. Vet J (London, England: 1997) 1998;155:189–95.

17. Pacheco AP, Paradis MR, Hoffman AM, et al. Age effects on blood gas, spirometry, airway reactivity, and bronchoalveolar lavage fluid cytology in clinically healthy horses. J Vet Intern Med 2014;28:603–8.

18. Hoffman AM, Kuehn H, Riedelberger K, et al. Flowmetric comparison of respiratory inductance plethysmography and pneumotachography in horses. J Appl Physiol 2001;91:2767–75.

19. Hoffman AM, Oura TJ, Riedelberger KJ, et al. Plethysmographic comparison of breathing pattern in heaves (recurrent airway obstruction) versus experimental bronchoconstriction or hyperpnea in horses. J Vet Intern Med 2007; 21:184–92.

20. Nolen-Walston RD, Kuehn H, Boston RC, et al. Reproducibility of airway responsiveness in horses using flowmetric plethysmography and histamine bronchoprovocation. J Vet Intern Med 2009;23:631–5.

21. Wichtel M, Gomez D, Burton S, et al. Relationships between equine airway reactivity measured by flowmetric plethysmography and specific indicators of airway inflammation in horses with suspected inflammatory airway disease. Equine Vet J 2015. [Epub ahead of print].

22. McFarlane D. Equine pituitary pars intermedia dysfunction. Vet Clin North Am Equine Pract 2011;27:93–113.

23. Mazan MR. Use of aerosolized bronchodilators and corticosteroids. In: Robinson NE, editor. Current therapy in equine medicine. Philadelphia: Saunders; 2003. p. 440–5.

24. Lavoie JP, Dalle S, Breton L, et al. Bronchiectasis in three adult horses with heaves. J Vet Intern Med 2004;18:757–60.
25. Johansson AM, Gardner SY, Atkins CE, et al. Cardiovascular effects of acute pulmonary obstruction in horses with recurrent airway obstruction. J Vet Intern Med 2007;21:302–7.
26. Davis JL, Gardner SY, Schwabenton B, et al. Congestive heart failure in horses: 14 cases (1984-2001). J Am Vet Med Assoc 2002;220:1512–5.
27. Sage AM, Valberg S, Hayden DW, et al. Echocardiography in a horse with cor pulmonale from recurrent airway obstruction. J Vet Intern Med 2006;20:694–6.
28. Hanka J, van den Hoven R, Schwarz B. Paroxysmal atrial fibrillation and clinically reversible cor pulmonale in a horse with complicated recurrent airway obstruction. Tierarztliche Praxis Ausgabe G Grosstiere Nutztiere 2015;43:109–14.
29. Glover CM, Miller LM, Dybdal NO, et al. Extrapituitary and pituitary pathological findings in horses with pituitary pars intermedia dysfunction: a retrospective study. J Equine Vet Sci 2009;29:146–53.
30. Else RW, Holmes JR. Cardiac pathology in the horse. 1. Gross pathology. Equine Vet J 1972;4:1–8.
31. Bishop S, Cole Cr, Smetzer DL. Functional and morphologic pathology of equine aortic insufficiency. Pathol Vet 1966;3:137–58.
32. Else R, Holmes JR. Cardiac pathology in the horse (2) Microscopic Pathology. Equine Vet J 1972;4:57–62.
33. Reef VB, Spencer P. Echocardiographic evaluation of equine aortic insufficiency. Am J Vet Res 1987;48:904–9.
34. Holmes JR. Equine cardiology, vol. 3. Bristol (United Kingdom): Langford; JR Homes; 1987.
35. Horn J. Sympathetic nervous control of cardiac function and its role in equine heart disease. Royal Veterinary College University of London; 2002.
36. Stadler P, Hoch M, Fraunhaul B, et al. Echocardiography in horses with and without heart murmurs in aortic regurgitation. Pferdeheikunde 1995;11:373–83.
37. Patteson MW. Echocardiographic evaluation of horses with aortic regurgitation. Equine Vet Educ 1994;6:159–66.
38. Horn J, Marr CM, Elliott J, et al. Identification of prognostic factors in equine aortic insufficiency. J Vet Intern Med 2002;16:335.
39. Miller P, Holmes JR. Observations on seven cases of mitral insufficiency in the horse. Equine Vet J 1985;17:181–90.
40. Reef VB, Bain FT, Spencer PA. Severe mitral regurgitation in horses: clinical, echocardiographic and pathological findings. Equine Vet J 1998;30:18–27.
41. Holmes J, Miller PJ. Three cases of ruptured mitral valve chordae in the horse. Equine Vet J 1984;16:125–35.
42. Reef VB. Advances in echocardiography. Vet Clin North Am Equine Pract 1991;7: 435–50.
43. Reef VB. Mitral valvular insufficiency associated with ruptured chordae tendineae in three foals. J Am Vet Med Assoc 1987;191:329–31.
44. Verheyen T, Decloedt A, van der Vekens N, et al. Ventricular response during lungeing exercise in horses with lone atrial fibrillation. Equine Vet J 2013;45:309–14.
45. Solis ND, Green C, Sides R, et al. Arrhythmias in Thoroughbreds during and after treadmill and racetrack exercise. Equine Vet J 2014;46:24–5.
46. Reef VB, Klumpp S, Maxson AD, et al. Echocardiographic detection of an intact aneurysm in a horse. J Am Vet Med Assoc 1990;197:752–5.
47. Rooney JR, Prickett ME, Crowe MW. Aortic ring rupture in stallions. Pathol Vet 1967;4:268–74.

48. Rooney JR. Rupture of the aorta. Mod Vet Pract 1979;60:391–2.
49. Sleeper MM, Durando MM, Miller M, et al. Aortic root disease in four horses. J Am Vet Med Assoc 2001;219:491–6.
50. Marr CM, Reef VB, Brazil TJ, et al. Aorto-cardiac fistulas in seven horses. Vet Radiol Ultrasound 1998;39:22–31.
51. Shirai W, Momotani E, Sato T, et al. Dissecting aortic aneurysm in a horse. J Comp Pathol 1999;120:307–11.
52. Lester G, Lombard CW, Ackerman N. Echocardiographic detection of a dissecting aortic root aneurysm in a Thoroughbred stallion. Vet Radiol Ultrasound 1992;33:202–5.
53. Roby KA, Reef VB, Shaw DP, et al. Rupture of an aortic sinus aneurysm in a 15-year-old broodmare. J Am Vet Med Assoc 1986;189:305–8.
54. Sweeney CR, Gillette DM. Thoracic neoplasia in equids: 35 cases (1967-1987). J Am Vet Med Assoc 1989;195:374–7.
55. Mair TS, Brown PJ. Clinical and pathological features of thoracic neoplasia in the horse. Equine Vet J 1993;25:220–3.
56. Knowles EJ, Tremaine WH, Pearson GR, et al. A database survey of equine tumours in the United Kingdom. Equine Vet J 2015;48(3):280–4.
57. Kelley LC, Hill JE, Hafner S, et al. Spontaneous equine pulmonary granular cell tumors: morphologic, histochemical, and immunohistochemical characterization. Vet Pathol 1995;32:101–6.
58. Goodchild LM, Dart AJ, Collins MB, et al. Granular cell tumour in the bronchus of a horse. Aust Vet J 1997;75:16–8.
59. Heinola T, Heikkila M, Ruohoniemi M, et al. Hypertrophic pulmonary osteopathy associated with granular cell tumour in a mare. Vet Rec 2001;149:307–8.
60. Ohnesorge B, Gehlen H, Wohlsein P. Transendoscopic electrosurgery of an equine pulmonary granular cell tumor. Vet Surg 2002;31:375–8.
61. Horn J, Bailey S, Berhane Y, et al. Density and binding characteristics of beta-adrenoceptors in the normal and failing equine myocardium. Equine Vet J 2002;34:411–6.
62. Koyak Z, Kroon B, de Groot JR, et al. Efficacy of antiarrhythmic drugs in adults with congenital heart disease and supraventricular tachycardias. Am J Cardiol 2013;112:1461–7.
63. Weeke P, Delaney J, Mosley JD, et al. QT variability during initial exposure to sotalol: experience based on a large electronic medical record. Europace 2013;15:1791–7.
64. Juvet T, Gourineni VC, Ravi S, et al. Life-threatening hyperkalemia: a potentially lethal drug combination. Conn Med 2013;77:491–3.
65. Gehlen H, Vieht JC, Stadler P. Effects of the ACE inhibitor quinapril on echocardiographic variables in horses with mitral valve insufficiency. J Vet Med A Physiol Pathol Clin Med 2003;50:460–5.
66. Gardner SY, Atkins CE, Sams RA, et al. Characterization of the pharmacokinetic and pharmacodynamic properties of the angiotensin-converting enzyme inhibitor, enalapril, in horses. J Vet Intern Med 2004;18:231–7.
67. Sleeper MM, McDonnell SM, Ely JJ, et al. Chronic oral therapy with enalapril in normal ponies. J Vet Cardiol 2008;10:111–5.
68. Afonso T, Giguere S, Rapoport G, et al. Cardiovascular effects of pimobendan in healthy mature horses. Equine Vet J 2016;45(3):352–6.
69. Freestone J, Carlson GP, Harrold DR, et al. Influence of furosemide treatment on fluid and electrolyte balance in the horse. Am J Vet Res 1988;49:1899–902.

Endocrine Disease in Aged Horses

Andy E. Durham, BSc, BVSc, CertEP, MRCVS

KEYWORDS

- Equine • Endocrine • PPID • EMS

KEY POINTS

- Aging may be associated with increased incidence of endocrinopathic conditions.
- Two foremost such problems, pituitary pars intermedia dysfunction and equine metabolic syndrome, merit consideration when indicative clinical signs are encountered in elderly horses.
- A few further minor endocrinopathies may occasionally be encountered, generally as a consequence of neoplasia of both endocrine and nonendocrine organs.

INTRODUCTION

Interest in both endocrine disease and geriatric health care has risen tremendously in recent years and is associated with a longer useful working life and an increasingly compassionate management approach with more retired horses being kept as companions. Pituitary pars intermedia dysfunction (PPID) is the best known and possibly the most common endocrinopathy in aged horses, although equine metabolic syndrome (EMS) is by no means uncommon. Indeed the 2 conditions may coexist. Consequently, discussion of PPID and EMS predominate in this article, with a little further discussion of rarer endocrinopathies.

PITUITARY PARS INTERMEDIA DYSFUNCTION
Definition and Pathophysiology

PPID remains relatively poorly understood with respect to its secretory products and their effects. The primary problem in PPID is thought to be neurodegeneration affecting inhibitory dopaminergic hypothalamic neurons and leading to hypertrophy, hyperplasia, and possibly microadenoma and macroadenoma development within the pars intermedia (PI) melanotrope cell population.[1] Increased concentrations of several immunoreactive peptides have been found, including α-melanocyte stimulating hormone, β-endorphin, corticotrophin-like immunoreactive peptide, and

Disclosure Statement: The author has nothing to disclose.
Liphook Equine Hospital, Liphook, Hampshire GU30 7JG, UK
E-mail address: andy.durham@theleh.co.uk

Vet Clin Equine 32 (2016) 301–315
http://dx.doi.org/10.1016/j.cveq.2016.04.007
0749-0739/16/$ – see front matter

adrenocorticotrophic hormone (ACTH),[2] although the precise consequences of these increased peptide concentrations are not well understood.

Along with a greater interest in PPID cases has come earlier clinical suspicion. Previous expectation of PPID cases were lethargic individuals demonstrating marked hypertrichosis along with recurrent laminitis, muscle wastage, a pendulous abdomen, and perhaps additional problems such as polydipsia, polyuria, recurrent infections, and abnormal sweating patterns most likely represented end-stage disease.[3,4] Indeed, short survival times were described and relatively high drug doses advised for treatment. An important development in recent years has been earlier recognition of disease. The clinical picture is frequently more subtle, including decreased athletic performance, loss of topline, mild attitude changes, hoof and laminar changes in the absence of obvious foot pain, and slightly delayed spring shedding and/or regional hypertrichosis.[5,6]

Diagnosis of Pituitary Pars Intermedia Dysfunction

Earlier investigation of disease has also brought diagnostic difficulties. Initial studies into laboratory diagnosis of PPID tended to find perfect dichotomy between normal and diseased populations, probably due to advanced endocrinopathy in the latter group.[7,8] Intuitively, earlier and milder disease may be harder to detect than when investigating advanced disease and, indeed, more recent studies indicate less impressive diagnostic sensitivity of PPID laboratory tests.[9,10]

Measurement of basal plasma ACTH concentration seems to be the most popular diagnostic test for investigation of PPID, perhaps due to the relative simplicity of collection of a single sample and seasonal reference intervals that allow testing at any time of year.[11] In normal horses, 98% of circulating ACTH is secreted from the pars distalis (PD),[12] whereas in PPID cases far higher amounts of PI-derived ACTH are released into the plasma.[12,13] Paradoxically, although higher measured plasma ACTH concentrations are clearly associated with the presence of PPID,[8] secondary adrenal hyperplasia is frequently absent and plasma total cortisol concentration is usually normal.[14–17] This may be explained by the PI-derived immunoreactive ACTH being significantly less bioactive than the PD-derived ACTH from normal horses.[13,17,18] Thus plasma ACTH in suspected PPID cases may be important diagnostically but less relevant physiologically.

Despite concerns regarding in vitro stability, plasma ACTH seems to be a good choice for PPID diagnosis in practice as long as plasma is chilled within 3 hours of collection and the sample remains chilled or frozen following centrifugation, until the time of processing.[6] Diagnosis of PPID based on plasma ACTH might intuitively be confounded by stressful events at the time of sampling or even the sampling procedure itself. Several studies have examined this possible effect and concluded that relatively mild pain, stress, and concurrent illness are unlikely to affect diagnostic usefulness of ACTH.[19–21] However, strenuous exercise, moderate to severe illness, and severe pain may all increase plasma ACTH[22,23] and when these conditions exist care should be taken in interpreting the results.

Since Donaldson and colleagues[24] first noted that plasma ACTH was significantly higher in healthy horses in September compared with January and May, further studies have better defined circannual variability, establishing seasonal reference intervals to enable year-round use of ACTH as a diagnostic test for PPID.[11] More recent data from a very large number of horses suggest the period of increased ACTH production is triggered by the summer solstice and extends between July and November inclusive with a peak in the last week of September.[25] It is also noteworthy that seasonal cues are retained in PPID, leading to especially high ACTH concentrations in PPID cases during the autumn.[11] Consistent with this, a more recent study demonstrated that the highest sensitivity and specificity of basal plasma ACTH for PPID diagnosis was in the autumn.[26]

The search for greater test sensitivity, at least during months outside of autumn, has produced interest in the thyrotropin-releasing hormone (TRH) stimulation test (**Box 1**), which generally seems to be a more accurate test than measurement of basal plasma ACTH alone.[9,10,17] Stimulation of TRH receptors present on both PI melanotropes and PD corticotrophs leads to increases in plasma ACTH in normal and PPID horses, although the response is significantly greater in PPID cases.

It is important to remember that dysinsulinemia is a common feature of PPID as well as EMS. Assessment of insulin-glucose dynamics is important as a predictor of laminitis, prognosis, and to guide dietary advice in PPID cases[6,28] (see later discussion of EMS for test details).

Management of Pituitary Pars Intermedia Dysfunction

Many related and unrelated comorbidities are frequently seen in PPID cases and should not be neglected while focusing on the endocrinopathy. Body condition should be assessed and dietary advice offered as appropriate. Changing social hierarchy should be considered as a contributor to weight loss as a result of aging or perhaps the behavioral effects of PPID. When horses are significantly underweight then investigation of additional causes related to PPID should be considered, including parasitism, diabetes mellitus (DM), chronic infections, and nonsteroidal antiinflammatory drug toxicity; as well as unrelated issues such as dental disease, liver disease, chronic renal failure, and so on.

Pergolide mesylate is the most popular therapeutic choice to reestablish the diminished dopaminergic control over the PI.[6] Treatment is typically initiated at 2 µg/kg every 24 hours with increased doses used if required.[6] Doses as high as 10 to 14 µg/kg have been reported,[4,29,30] although anorexia is likely at higher doses and is occasionally reported at lower doses too.[31]

Clinical response can be evaluated after 1 to 3 months based on start of hair shedding, improvement of laminitis and general attitude, increasing activity, and a decrease in water consumption if previously polydipsic.[31–36] Additionally, monitoring changes in laboratory indicators of PPID may offer a more objective and more sensitive means of assessing response to treatment, especially when less predictable clinical signs such as laminitis exist. However, changes in clinical and laboratory indicators of PPID do not always concur, which may create dilemmas in ongoing management and treatment decisions. Although clinical improvement is clearly reassuring, continued abnormally high plasma ACTH (or other endocrine test result) is direct evidence of ongoing pituitary dysfunction.

Box 1
Protocol for thyrotropin-releasing hormone stimulation test

- Collect plasma for basal ACTH measurement
- Inject 1 mg TRH intravenously
- Collect further plasma samples for ACTH at 10 and/or 30 minutes later
- Cut-offs of 110 pg/mL and 65 pg/mL, respectively, are suggested[27]
- Lack of valid reference intervals means that this test should not be used between July and November inclusive

Several studies have documented improvement in laboratory variables, including basal ACTH following treatment with pergolide.[31–36] In a study of 113 PPID cases, improvement in clinical signs and endocrine test results was observed in 76% of cases following treatment with pergolide for 180 days.[31] It is suggested that at least 4 weeks of pergolide treatment be given before considering dosage increases,[6,27] although good treatment responses can be delayed for as long as 3 to 4 years in some cases (H.C. Schott, personal communication, 2016), perhaps depending on the nature of the underlying PI pathologic state. It is not currently known whether it is longer duration of treatment or increased doses of pergolide that play a primary role in initial nonresponders that later come under endocrine control.

Ongoing monitoring of PPID cases is important to discuss with the owner due to the potentially progressive nature of the endocrinopathy itself, as well as the likelihood of further morbidities developing in aged horses. It is generally recommended that PPID cases should be monitored both clinically and endocrinologically at least twice per annum, with 1 recheck being scheduled within the period of circannual increase in pituitary activity.[6,27]

EQUINE METABOLIC SYNDROME
Definition and Pathophysiology

EMS could be described as a collection of commonly coexisting risk factors, associated with metabolic and endocrine dysregulation that signal an increased susceptibility to laminitis. Cases tend to be from certain breed types, often obese and demonstrating dysregulation of insulin-glucose dynamics as well as disordered lipid metabolism (dysinsulinemia).

Generous feeding and management practices in rather sedentary populations of genetically susceptible horses, ponies, and donkeys have led to frequent clinical encounters with EMS cases. A metabolically efficient phenotype, known as easy-keepers or good-doers, typifies EMS cases.[37] Aging may often result in continuation or progression of EMS, perhaps due to decreased energy demands associated with reduced athletic activities and well-intentioned increased dietary provision for older horses. Thus, EMS is a genuine problem in elderly horses and should be considered with equal prominence alongside PPID when laminitis in seen in such individuals. Indeed, these 2 endocrinopathies are by no means mutually exclusive and can coexist in the same individual.

Laminitis seems to be the main morbidity associated with EMS, although other problems such as hyperlipemia, lethargy, and infertility have been purported also. The roots of understanding of what is now known as EMS actually began in the 1980s,[38] although the relevance and importance of the condition was not realized widely before the description by Johnson[39] in 2002.

Dysinsulinemia currently seems central to the pathophysiology and diagnosis of EMS.[40–42] It is possible that dysinsulinemia may arise from a basis of genetic determinants on which are superimposed additional acquired influences, such as diet and obesity, which then lead to pathologic consequences.[40] It is plausible that natural selection may have promoted evolution of changes in insulin metabolism in surroundings where nutritional supply was sparse and/or inconsistently present. Resistance to the endocrine effects of insulin would tend to preserve scarce glucose for use in vital noninsulin-dependent tissues such as the central nervous system, renal tissue, and cardiac muscle. Furthermore, it would facilitate gluconeogenesis and the mobilization of glycogen and fat stores when required at times of limited food supply (eg, after snowfall or during drought), offering a survival advantage. It may also be the case that pancreatic beta cells developed lower secretory thresholds for synthesis and release of insulin in cases in which the typical diet lacked much stimulus for insulin secretion. Thus, evolutionary pressures may have led to relative insulin resistance and low secretory threshold for insulin release, promoting gene establishment and improved survival of certain individuals and certain breeds in nutritionally harsh environments.

Acquired dysinsulinemia has been demonstrated following development of obesity following overfeeding with high nonstructural carbohydrate (NSC) feeds.[43,44] Thus, possible genetic determinants of dysinsulinemia may be magnified by further acquired dietary or obesity effects associated with modern domestication in which equids are effectively protected against the harsh nutritional environment in which their ancestors may have evolved. Consequences of this pathologic chronic dysinsulinemia and maintenance of adipose stores seem to include risk of hyperlipemia with sudden and precipitous lipid catabolism,[45] and increased risk of laminitis.[37,42]

Laminitis is triggered predictably in normal horses and ponies by exposing them to hyperinsulinemia for 48 hours,[46–48] suggesting that hyperinsulinemia may be the link between dysinsulinemia and laminitis. Postprandial hyperinsulinemia is a consequence of consuming high NSC feeds[49,50] but the magnitude and duration of hyperinsulinemia is often exaggerated in individuals with dysinsulinemia, creating a greater probability of suprathreshold pathogenic hyperinsulinemia precipitating laminitis development in predisposed horses.[50,51]

Diagnosis of Equine Metabolic Syndrome

Many potential supportive tests exist when investigating the possibility of EMS and they can be considered logically in related but distinct categories or tiers as tests that identify

1. Dysinsulinemia
   a. A tendency towards hyperinsulinemia, the direct cause of laminitis
   b. Insulin resistance, a promoter of hyperinsulinemia (1a)
2. Risk factors for insulin resistance (1b), including obesity and adipokines.

Hyperinsulinemia tests

The primary importance of a tendency towards excessive postprandial hyperinsulinemia can be investigated by using oral sugar challenge tests, including corn syrup, dextrose, or glucose[42,52,53] (**Boxes 2** and **3**). Abnormal test results demonstrating excessive hyperinsulinemia imply a similar response might follow ingestion of grazing or cereal feeds, placing that individual at higher risk of diet-induced laminitis.

Box 2
The corn syrup oral sugar test

- Fast for at least 5 to 6 hours (allow a small amount of hay the previous night)
- Administer 0.15 mL/kg Karo Light Corn Syrup
- Measure plasma insulin between 60 to 90 minutes later
- An excessive insulin response is defined by insulin greater than 60 mU/L (suspicious when > 45 mu/L)

Data from Schuver A, Frank N, Chameroy KA, Elliot SB Assessment of insulin and glucose dynamics using an oral sugar test in horses. J Equine Vet Sci 2014;34:465–70.

Box 3
The glucose or dextrose oral sugar test

- Fast for at least 5 to 6 hours (allow a small amount of hay the previous night)
- Administer 1 g/kg glucose or dextrose powder in a small feed of chopped hay or straw (or other low-NSC feed)
- Measure plasma glucose and insulin 120 minutes later
- An excessive insulin response is defined by insulin greater than 85 mU/L (A.E. Durham, unpublished data, 2010)
- Plasma glucose less than 7.5 mmol/L suggests an invalid test with poor consumption and/or absorption of the test dose

---

Testing insulin resistance Although hyperinsulinemia may be the direct pathologic instigator of laminitis, supporting the diagnostic usefulness of oral sugar tests, additional tests examining the effectiveness of insulin may be diagnostically useful because insulin resistance promotes hyperinsulinemia. Many methods exist for examining insulin resistance in horses, although few are practical for use outside of a laboratory setting.[42] Simple resting hypertriglyceridemia implies insulin resistance, although abnormalities tend to be relatively subtle in EMS cases.[40] The 2-step insulin-response test[54] is perhaps the simplest dynamic test for use in practice and can be used to estimate the presence and degree of insulin resistance, and to then monitor changes in insulin sensitivity following management improvements (**Box 4**).

Measuring risk factors for insulin resistance
In addition to genetic determinants, acquired insulin resistance is a consequence of chronically excessive caloric provision.[43,44] Objective and semiobjective measures of consequent obesity are relevant to EMS diagnosis and monitoring, including morphologic scoring systems such as body condition score[40,55] and cresty neck score.[41,56] Although well validated, such measures may be insensitive for detecting significant weight loss and improved insulin sensitivity.[57] Objective morphologic measurements such as girth to height ratio or neck circumference to height ratio are attractive but do not seem to perform as well as the aforementioned semiobjective scoring

---

Box 4
Details of the 2-step insulin-response test

- No fasting required; allow hay access
- Measure baseline plasma glucose
- Inject 0.1 mU/kg regular insulin intravenously
- Measure plasma glucose at 30 minutes
- In normal horses plasma glucose is expected to decrease by at least 50% at 30 minutes
- Smaller decreases indicate insulin resistance.
- Monitor for signs of hypoglycemia for 60 minutes and/or inject 30 mL/100 kg 50% glucose intravenously after collection of the 30-minute sample

Data from Bertin FR, Sojka-Kritchevsky JE. Comparison of a 2-step insulin-response test to conventional insulin-sensitivity testing in horses. Domest Anim Endocrinol 2013;44:19–25.

---

methods.[56] Additionally, evidence suggests that increased adiposity is not always associated with dysinsulinemia.[44]

In common parlance, obesity tends to be regarded as a morphologic term related to quantity of adipose tissue. However, the term actually implies a condition in which excess body fat has accumulated to the extent that it may have an adverse effect on health and is, therefore, strictly a functional or qualitative, rather than simply a morphologic or quantitative, term. It is perfectly plausible that individuals with a sparse amount of more highly pathogenic adipose tissue are actually more obese than individuals with larger amounts of benign adipose deposits.[58] Thus, functional measures of obesity might prove to be better indicators of EMS, including measurement of a variety of adipose-derived endocrine products known as adipokines.[59] In horses, the 2 best investigated adipokines are leptin and adiponectin, which have been found to be abnormally increased and decreased, respectively, in association with obesity.[60] Current evidence favors adiponectin as a better indicator of the functional effects of excessive adiposity[44,61,62] and metabolic improvement in association with weight loss programs.[63] Although reference intervals have not yet been well established in horses, experiences indicate that most normal individuals with have high molecular weight adiponectin values greater than 3 to 4 μg/mL.[62,64]

Management of Equine Metabolic Syndrome

Invariably, EMS results from caloric excess with respect to energy expenditure and, therefore, should be tackled fundamentally by restoring this imbalance. This solution is frequently challenging in individuals with tremendous metabolic efficiency, and sometimes chronic laminitis, that limits exercise capability. However, many excellent studies have now been conducted to better inform effective ration control, enabling successful weight loss in the hands of motivated and determined owners[65] (**Box 5**).

Medical support of EMS cases has been described with levothyroxine[67] and metformin.[68] These products may play a useful role in some cases, especially those in which management interventions are suboptimal. The potential limiting effect of metformin on postprandial hyperinsulinemia is particularly interesting in the light of the previously described pathophysiologic events determining laminitis causation.[69,70]

OTHER ENDOCRINOPATHIES

Other than PPID and EMS, other endocrinopathic conditions are uncommon to rare in horses. A few of these seem to be associated with aging and are discussed briefly.

Diseases Affecting Glucose Homeostasis

Diabetes mellitus
Diabetes mellitus (DM) is defined as persistent hyperglycemia resulting from defects in insulin secretion, insulin action, or both. The most common clinical presentation is

---

Box 5
Summary of key points in ration formulation for equine metabolic syndrome cases

- Eliminate (or at least greatly restrict) grazing, cereal, or other insulinemic dietary sources
- Feed low NSC (<10–12%) forage between 1.0% to 2.0% of bodyweight daily (as fed)
- Hay soaking can be used to reduce water-soluble carbohydrate content (but the additional effect of soaking on loss of further key nutrients should not be underestimated[66]
- Ration balancers added to ensure adequate protein and micronutrient intake

weight loss, polydipsia, and polyuria. Laboratory findings necessarily include hyperglycemia (confirmed on more than 1 occasion), although insulin concentration can be high, low, or normal, depending on the type and stage of DM. Hypertriglyceridemia is also frequently seen and unexpected grossly evident lipemia is an important indicator of DM in horses. High plasma fructosamine helps confirm chronicity of hyperglycemia. Glycosuria is generally, although not invariably, present because this depends on the magnitude of hyperglycemia and whether or not it exceeds the renal threshold.

Most cases of DM in aging horses are probably associated with PPID and are assumed to represent type 2 DM given the evidence of insulin resistance associated with many cases of PPID.[71] Although type 2 DM is reported in association with suspected EMS, it is a relatively rare consequence in comparison with the almost inevitable development of type 2 diabetes in obese humans.[52]

Dietary management of DM should comprise a ration of low NSC feed content with free access to grass hay alongside feeds of good quality fermentable fiber such as beet pulp that has not been molassed, coconut meal, or almond hulls. Therapy for DM in horses is most effective in cases in which there is a treatable underlying condition. One report indicated a rapid resolution of chronic hyperglycemia following pergolide therapy in a horse with PPID.[71] Attempted exogenous insulin therapy has been described several times in the literature but is challenging given the expense and difficulties in case management. However, in rare cases of type 1 DM there may be few other drugs that are likely to be helpful so insulin therapy might be considered.[72] In cases of type 2 DM that are not responsive to pergolide, then drugs which stimulate further endogenous insulin secretion, such as glyburide (glibenclamide), have been reported.[71]

Neoplasia-associated hypoglycemia

Insulinoma, a pancreatic beta-cell neoplasm characterized by uncontrolled insulin secretion and consequent hypoglycemia, seems to be extremely rare in horses with only 1 reported case in a Shetland pony suffering recurrent seizures.[73] Hypoglycemia has also been reported several times in horses with nonislet cell tumors, including hepatic,[74,75] renal,[76,77] mesothelial,[78] and gastric[79] neoplasia. Clinical signs of ataxia, weakness, blindness, mental obtundation, excessive sweating, seizures, and muscular tremors are reported. Although insulin-like growth factors are a cause of similar disease in other species, this remains speculative in horses.[77]

Thyroid Disorders

Unilateral thyroid masses are commonly encountered in aging horses and generally represent nonfunctional C-cell adenomas.[80] Primary dysfunctional thyroid disease seems to be very rare in horses.

Hypothyroidism

Clinical suspicion of primary hypothyroidism should be considered in the context of the subtle clinical effects of total thyroidectomy in horses, which may lead to little more than a coarse hair coat and cold intolerance.[81] Reduced thyroid secretory activity, when it does occur in horses, is most likely to be secondary to other factors, such as coexisting nonthyroidal illness or drug treatment (eg, phenylbutazone), rather than primary thyroidal disease.[82]

Normal or high resting concentrations of total or free triiodothyronine (T3) and thyroxine (T4) are not compatible with a diagnosis of hypothyroidism but low concentrations are certainly not confirmatory. Thyroid hormone response at 2 and 4 hours following 1 mg TRH intravenous (**Table 1**) is a reasonably simple functional

Table 1
Expected hormone response to 1 mg thyrotropin-releasing hormone intravenous demonstrating mean and range of increases expected

Hormone Assayed	0–2 h Response		0–4 h Response	
	Mean	Range	Mean	Range
Total T3	3 ×	(1.1–10.3 ×)	—	—
Free T3	4.2 ×	(1–53 ×)	—	—
Total T4	—	—	2.2 ×	(1.3–3.8 ×)
Free T4	—	—	1.7 ×	(1.1–2.1 ×)
Free T4 by dialysis	—	—	1.8 ×	(1.1–2.8 ×)

Horses with low responses tended to have either higher resting values or had peaks at different times than 2 or 4 hours.

Data from Breuhaus BA. Disorders of the equine thyroid gland. Vet Clin North Am Equine Pract 2011;27:115–28.

test of the thyroid axis[83] and can be used to investigate suspected hypothyroid cases.

Hyperthyroidism

Hyperthyroidism is rare, although a few well-described reports exist of endocrinologically active thyroid tumors resulting in weight loss, hyperactivity, and unilateral thyroid enlargement in elderly horses.[83–86] Hyperthyroidism is best diagnosed by using a T3 suppression test whereby T4 is measured following multiple injections of exogenous T3 over a few days.[85] An autonomously active thyroid gland will continue to produce high levels of T4 despite exogenous T3. Treatment may be medical or surgical.[83–86]

Hyperparathyroidism

Primary hyperparathyroidism due to functional parathyroid adenoma is occasionally reported in aging horses, leading to weight loss, depression, anorexia, and shifting lameness.[87,88] A combination of hypercalcemia and high plasma parathyroid hormone (PTH) concentration is suggestive. Effective treatment comprises parathyroidectomy, although the location of the glands can be difficult to identify.[89,90]

Hypercalcemia of malignancy is a separate disorder in which PTH-related peptide (PTHrp), or possibly other hypercalcemic cytokines, may be secreted from tumors, including lymphoma, myeloma, and squamous cell carcinoma.[91,92] Specific clinical signs are often lacking because the presentation is often dominated by underlying neoplasia. Nevertheless, unexplained hypercalcemia should alert the clinician to this possibility.

Adrenal Disorders

Adrenal cortex

Both hypoadrenocorticism and hyperadrenocorticism are rare conditions in horses. Despite frequent assumption to the contrary, several studies indicate that hyperadrenocorticism is not a common consequence of PPID in horses.[13–18] There is only a single well-described case of functional adrenocortical adenoma in a horse, which resulted in ravenous appetite, muscle wasting, bulging supraorbital fat, delayed shedding of the coat, hyperhidrosis, and lethargy.[93]

Adrenal medulla

Pheochromocytomas are neoplasms of the chromaffin cells of the adrenal medulla and are occasionally encountered in horses, sometimes alongside other endocrine diseases as part of a syndrome of multiple endocrine neoplasia.[94,95] Nonfunctional tumors are reported as incidental findings post mortem.[95] However, when functional, they secrete excessive quantities of catecholamines and usually result in signs of colic.[94,96] It is possible that a perirenal mass may be palpable or ultrasonographically imageable. Peritoneal fluid is frequently hemorrhagic and blood tests often reflect polycythemia, azotemia, and hypergylcemia.[94,96]

REFERENCES

1. Miller MA, Pardo ID, Jackson LP, et al. Correlation of pituitary histomorphometry with adrenocorticotrophic hormone response to domperidone administration in the diagnosis of equine pituitary pars intermedia dysfunction. Vet Pathol 2008; 45:26–38.

2. Millington WR, Dybdal NO, Dawson R, et al. Equine Cushing's disease: differential regulation of beta-endorphin processing in tumors of the intermediate pituitary. Endocrinology 1988;123:1598–604.

3. Beech J. Tumors of the pituitary gland (pars intermedia). In: Robinson NE, editor. Current therapy in equine medicine. 1st edition. Philadelphia: W.B. Saunders; 1983. p. 164–8.

4. Beech J. Tumors of the pituitary gland (pars intermedia). In: Robinson NE, editor. Current therapy in equine medicine. 3rd edition. Philadelphia: W.B. Saunders; 1987. p. 182–5.

5. McGowan TW, Pinchbeck GP, McGowan CM. Prevalence, risk factors and clinical signs predictive for equine pituitary pars intermedia dysfunction in aged horses. Equine Vet J 2013;45:74–9.

6. Durham A, McGowan C, Fey K, et al. The diagnosis and treatment of PPID in the horse. Equine Vet Educ 2014;26:216–23.

7. Dybdal NO, Hargreaves KM, Madigan JE, et al. Diagnostic testing for pituitary pars intermedia dysfunction in horses. J Am Vet Med Assoc 1994;204:627–32.

8. van der Kolk JH, Wensing T, Kalsbeek HC, et al. Laboratory diagnosis of equine pituitary pars intermedia adenoma. Domest Anim Endocrinol 1995;12:35–9.

9. Beech J, Boston R, Lindborg S, et al. Adrenocorticotropin concentration following administration of thyrotropin-releasing hormone in healthy horses and those with pituitary pars intermedia dysfunction and pituitary gland hyperplasia. J Am Vet Med Assoc 2007;231:417–26.

10. Beech J, McFarlane D, Lindborg S, et al. α-Melanocyte–stimulating hormone and adrenocorticotropin concentrations in response to thyrotropin-releasing hormone and comparison with adrenocorticotropin concentration after domperidone administration in healthy horses and horses with pituitary pars intermedia dysfunction. J Am Vet Med Assoc 2011;238:1305–15.

11. Copas VE, Durham AE. Circannual variation in plasma adrenocorticotropic hormone concentrations in the UK in normal horses and ponies, and those with pituitary pars intermedia dysfunction. Equine Vet J 2012;44:440–3.

12. Wilson MG, Nicholson WE, Holscher MA, et al. Proopiolipomelanocortin peptides in normal pituitary, pituitary tumor, and plasma of normal and Cushing's horse. Endocrinology 1982;110:941–54.

13. Orth DN, Nicholson WE. Bioactive and immunoreactive adrenocorticotropin in normal equine pituitary and in pituitary tumors of horses with Cushing's disease. Endocrinology 1982;111:559–63.

14. Heinrichs M, Baumgärtner W, Capen CC. Immunocytochemical demonstration of proopiomelanocortin-derived peptides in pituitary adenomas of the pars intermedia in horses. Vet Pathol 1990;27:419–25.

15. McFarlane D, Beech J, Cribb A. Alpha-melanocyte stimulating hormone release in response to thyrotropin releasing hormone in healthy horses, horses with pituitary pars intermedia dysfunction and equine pars intermedia explants. Domest Anim Endocrinol 2006;30:276–88.

16. Ellenberger C, Dolken M, Uhlig A, et al. Tumoren des endokriniums beim pferde – klinische pathologie. Pferdeheilkunde 2010;26:764–74.

17. Beech J, Boston R, Lindborg S. Comparison of cortisol and ACTH responses after administration of thyrotropin releasing hormone in normal horses and those with pituitary pars intermedia dysfunction. J Vet Intern Med 2011;25:1431–8.

18. Sommer K. Das Equine Cushing-Syndrom: Entwicklung eines ACTH-Bioassays für die Ermittlung des biologisch-immunreaktiven Verhältnisses von endogenem ACTH in equinen Blutproben. Inaugural dissertation to obtain the degree of doctor of veterinary medicine (Dr. med. vet.). University of Veterinary Medicine Hannover; 2003. Available at: http://elib.tiho-hannover.de/dissertations/sommerk_2003.pdf.

19. Alexander SL, Irvine CH, Livesey JH, et al. Effect of isolation stress on concentrations of arginine vasopressin, alpha-melanocyte-stimulating hormone and ACTH in the pituitary venous effluent of the normal horse. J Endocrinol 1988;116:325–34.

20. Couëtil L, Paradis MR, Knoll J. Plasma adrenocorticotropin concentration in healthy horses and in horses with clinical signs of hyperadrenocorticism. J Vet Intern Med 1996;10:1–6.

21. Fouché N, van der Kolk JH, Bruckmaier RM, et al. Venipuncture does not affect adrenocorticotropic hormone concentration in horses. Vet Rec 2015;177:223–4.

22. Alexander SL, Irvine CH, Ellis MJ, et al. The effect of acute exercise on the secretion of corticotropin-releasing factor, arginine vasopressin, and adrenocorticotropin as measured in pituitary venous blood from the horse. Endocrinology 1991;128:65–72.

23. Towns TJ, Stewart AJ, Hackett E, et al. Cortisol and ACTH concentrations in ill horses throughout 6 days of hospitalisation. J Vet Emerg Crit Care 2010;20:A16–7.

24. Donaldson MT, McDonnell SM, Schanbacher BJ, et al. Variation in plasma adrenocorticotropic hormone concentration and dexamethasone suppression test results with season, age, and sex in healthy ponies and horses. J Vet Intern Med 2005;19:217–22.

25. Durham A. Further Observations of Seasonality of Pars Intermedia Secretory Function in 30,000 Horses and Ponies. Proceedings of Dorothy Russell Havemeyer Foundation Equine Geriatric Workshop II, 3rd Equine Endocrine Summit. Middleburg (Virginia); November 17-20, 2014. Available at: https://sites.tufts.edu/equineendogroup/files/2013/10/Equine-Geriatric-Workshop-II-DRH-2014.pdf. Accessed May 4, 2016.

26. McGowan TW, Pinchbeck GP, McGowan CM. Evaluation of basal plasma a-melanocyte-stimulating hormone and adrenocorticotrophic hormone concentrations for the diagnosis of pituitary pars intermedia dysfunction from a population of aged horses. Equine Vet J 2013;45:66–73.

27. Frank N, Andrews F, Durham A, et al. Recommendations for the Diagnosis and Treatment of Pituitary Pars Intermedia Dysfunction (PPID). 2013. Available at: http://sites.tufts.edu/equineendogroup/. Accessed May 4, 2016.

28. McGowan CM, Frost R, Pfeiffer DU, et al. Serum insulin concentrations in horses with equine Cushing's syndrome: response to a cortisol inhibitor and prognostic value. Equine Vet J 2004;36:295–8.

29. Orth DN, Holscher MA, Wilson MG, et al. Equine Cushing's disease: plasma immunoreactive proopiolipomelanocortin peptide and cortisol levels basally and in response to diagnostic tests. Endocrinology 1982;110:1430–41.

30. Beech J. Treatment of hypophysial adenomas. Comp Cont Educ Pract Vet 1994; 16:921–3.

31. Andrews FM, McFarlane D, Stokes AM, et al. Freedom of information summary. Prascend Tablets, Pergolide Mesylate, for the control of clinical signs associated with Pituitary Pars Intermedia Dysfunction (Equine Cushing's Disease) in horses. Original New Animal Drug Application. NADA; 2011. p. 141–331. Available at: http://fda.gov/downloads/AnimalVeterinary/Products/ Approved AnimalDrug Products/FOIADrugSummaries/UCM280354.pdf.

32. Schott HC, Coursen CL, Eberhart SW, et al. The Michigan Cushing's Project. Proc AAEP 2001;47:22–4.

33. Donaldson MT, LaMonte BH, Morresey P, et al. Treatment with pergolide or cyproheptadine of pituitary pars intermedia dysfunction (Equine Cushing's Disease). J Vet Intern Med 2002;16:742–6.

34. Perkins GA, Lamb S, Erb HN, et al. Plasma adrenocorticotropin (ACTH) concentrations and clinical response in horses treated for equine Cushing's disease with cyproheptadine or pergolide. Equine Vet J 2002;34:679–85.

35. Pongratz MC, Graubner C, Eser MW. Equine Cushing's Syndrome. The effects of long-term therapy with pergolide. Pferdeheilkunde 2010;26:598–603.

36. Rohrbach BW, Stafford JR, Clermont RSW, et al. Diagnostic frequency, response to therapy, and long-term prognosis among horses and ponies with pituitary par intermedia dysfunction, 1993–2004. J Vet Intern Med 2012;26:1027–34.

37. Frank N, Geor RJ, Bailey SR, et al. Equine metabolic syndrome. J Vet Intern Med 2010;24:467–75.

38. Coffman JR, Colles CM. Insulin tolerance in laminitic ponies. Can J Comp Med 1983;47:347–51.

39. Johnson PJ. The equine metabolic syndrome: peripheral Cushing's syndrome. Vet Clin North Am Equine Pract 2002;18:271–93.

40. Treiber KH, Kronfeld DS, Hess TM, et al. Evaluation of genetic and metabolic predispositions and nutritional risk factors for pasture-associated laminitis in ponies. J Am Vet Med Assoc 2006;228:1538–45.

41. Carter RA, Geor RJ, Burton Staniar W, et al. Prediction of incipient pasture-associated laminitis from hyperinsulinemia, hyperleptinaemia and generalised and localised obesity in a cohort of ponies. Equine Vet J 2009;41:171–8.

42. Frank N, Tadros EM. Insulin dysregulation. Equine Vet J 2014;46:103–12.

43. Carter RA, McCutcheon LJ, George LA, et al. Effects of diet-induced weight gain on insulin sensitivity and plasma hormone and lipid concentrations in horses. Am J Vet Res 2009;70:1250–8.

44. Bamford NJ, Potter SJ, Baskerville CL, et al. Effect of increased adiposity of insulin sensitivity and adipokines concentrations in different equine breeds adapted to cereal rich and fat rich meals. Vet J 2016, in press.

45. Durham AE. Hyperlipemia. In: Coenen M, Harris P, Geor R, editors. Equine applied and clinical nutrition. Elsevier London; 2013. p. 512–20.

46. Asplin KE, Sillence MN, Pollitt CC, et al. Induction of laminitis by prolonged hyperinsulinemia in clinically normal ponies. Vet J 2007;174:530–5.

47. de Laat MA, McGowan CM, Sillence MN, et al. Equine laminitis: induced by 48 h hyperinsulinemia in Standardbred horses. Equine Vet J 2010;42:129–35.

48. de Laat MA, Sillence MN, McGowan CM, et al. Continuous intravenous infusion of glucose induces endogenous hyperinsulinemia and lamellar histopathology in Standardbred horses. Vet J 2012;191:317–22.

49. Coenen M, Mößeler A, Vervuert I. Fermentative gases in breath indicate that inulin and starch start to be degraded by microbial fermentation in the stomach and small intestine of the horse in contrast to pectin and cellulose. J Nutr 2006;136: 2108S–10S.

50. Borer KE, Bailey SR, Menzies-Gow NJ, et al. Effect of feeding glucose, fructose, and inulin on blood glucose and insulin concentrations in normal ponies and those predisposed to laminitis. J Anim Sci 2012;90:3003–11.

51. Tinworth KD, Raidal SL, Harris PA, et al. Comparing glycaemic and insulinemic responses of ponies and horses to dietary glucose (abstract). J Equine Vet Sci 2011;31:301.

52. Frank N. Equine metabolic syndrome. Vet Clin North Am Equine Pract 2011;27: 73–92.

53. Schuver A, Frank N, Chameroy KA, et al. Assessment of insulin and glucose dynamics using an oral sugar test in horses. J Equine Vet Sci 2014;34:465–70.

54. Bertin FR, Sojka-Kritchevsky JE. Comparison of a 2-step insulin-response test to conventional insulin-sensitivity testing in horses. Domest Anim Endocrinol 2013; 44:19–25.

55. Henneke DR, Potter GD, Kreider JL, et al. Relationship between condition score, physical measurement and body fat percentage in mares. Equine Vet J 1983;15: 371–2.

56. Carter RA, Geor RJ, Burton Staniar W, et al. Apparent adiposity assessed by standardised scoring systems and morphometric measurements in horses and ponies. Vet J 2009;179:204–10.

57. Dugdale AH, Curtis GC, Cripps P, et al. Effect of dietary restriction on body condition, composition and welfare of overweight and obese pony mares. Equine Vet J 2010;42:600–10.

58. Conus F, Rabasa-Lhoret R, Péronnet F. Characteristics of metabolically obese normal-weight (MONW) subjects. Appl Physiol Nutr Metab 2007;32:4–12.

59. Radin MJ, Sharkey LC, Holycross BJ. Adipokines: a review of biological and analytical principles and an update in dogs, cats, and horses. Vet Clin Pathol 2009;38:136–56.

60. Kearns CF, McKeever KH, Roegner V, et al. Adiponectin and leptin are related to fat mass in horses. Vet J 2006;172:460–5.

61. Gordon ME, McKeever KH, Betros CL, et al. Plasma leptin, ghrelin and adiponectin concentrations in young fit racehorses versus mature unfit standardbreds. Vet J 2007;173:91–100.

62. Bamford NJ, Potter SJ, Harris PA, et al. Effect of increased adiposity on insulin sensitivity and adipokine concentrations in horses and ponies fed a high fat diet, with or without a once daily high glycaemic meal. Equine Vet J 2016; 48(3):368–73.

63. Ungru J, Blüher M, Coenen M, et al. Effects of body weight reduction on blood adipokines and subcutaneous adipose tissue adipokine mRNA expression profiles in obese ponies. Vet Rec 2012;171:528–34.

64. Wooldridge AA, Edwards HG, Plaisance EP, et al. Evaluation of high-molecular weight adiponectin in horses. Am J Vet Res 2012;73:1230–40.

65. Geor RJ, Harris PA. Obesity. In: Coenen M, Harris P, Geor R, editors. Equine applied and clinical nutrition. Elsevier London; 2013. p. 487–502.
66. Argo CM, Dugdale AH, McGowan CM. Considerations for the use of restricted, soaked grass hay diets to promote weight loss in the management of equine metabolic syndrome and obesity. Vet J 2015;206(2):170–7.
67. Frank N, Elliott SB, Boston RC. Effects of long-term oral administration of levothyroxine sodium on glucose dynamics in healthy adult horses. Am J Vet Res 2008; 69:76–81.
68. Durham AE, Rendle DI, Newton JR. The effect of metformin on measurements of insulin sensitivity and beta cell response in 18 horses and ponies with insulin resistance. Equine Vet J 2008;40:493–500.
69. Durham AE. Metformin in equine metabolic syndrome: an enigma or a dead duck? Vet J 2012;191:17–8.
70. Rendle DI, Rutledge F, Hughes KJ, et al. Effects of metformin hydrochloride on blood glucose and insulin responses to oral dextrose in horses. Equine Vet J 2013;45:751–4.
71. Durham AE, Hughes KJ, Cottle HJ, et al. Type 2 diabetes mellitus with pancreatic beta cell dysfunction in 3 horses confirmed with minimal model analysis. Equine Vet J 2009;41:924–9.
72. Giri JK, Magdesian KG, Gaffney PM. Insulin-dependent diabetes mellitus associated with presumed autoimmune polyendocrine syndrome in a mare. Can Vet J 2011;52:506–12.
73. Ross MW, Lowe JE, Cooper BJ, et al. Hypoglycemic seizures in a Shetland pony. Cornell Vet 1983;73:151–69.
74. Roby K-AW, Beech J, Bloom JC, et al. Hepatocellular carcinoma associated with erythrocytosis and hypoglycemia in a yearling filly. J Am Vet Med Assoc 1990; 196:465–7.
75. Wong D, Hepworth K, Yaeger M, et al. Imaging diagnosis-hypoglycemia associated with cholangiocarcinoma and peritoneal carcinomatosis in a horse. Vet Radiol Ultrasound 2015;56:E9–12.
76. Baker JL, Aleman M, Madigan J. Intermittent hypoglycemia in a horse with anaplastic carcinoma of the kidney. J Am Vet Med Assoc 2001;218:235–7.
77. Swain JM, Pirie RS, Hudson NPH, et al. Insulin-like growth factors and recurrent hypoglycemia associated with renal cell carcinoma in a horse. J Vet Intern Med 2005;19:613–6.
78. LaCarrubba AM, Johnson PJ, Whitney MS, et al. Hypoglycemia and tumor lysis syndrome associated with peritoneal mesothelioma in a horse. J Vet Intern Med 2006;20:1018–22.
79. Haga HA, Ytrehus B, Rudshaug IJ, et al. Gastrointestinal stromal tumor and hypoglycemia in a Fjord pony: case report. Acta Vet Scand 2008;50:9–13.
80. Ueki H, Kowatari Y, Oyamada T, et al. Non-functional C-cell adenoma in aged horses. J Comp Pathol 2004;131:157–65.
81. Frank N, Sojka J. Messer NT equine thyroid dysfunction. Vet Clin North Am Equine Pract 2002;18:305–19.
82. Hilderbran AC, Breuhaus BA, Refsal KR. Nonthyroidal illness syndrome in adult horses. J Vet Intern Med 2014;28:609–17.
83. Breuhaus BA. Disorders of the equine thyroid gland. Vet Clin North Am Equine Pract 2011;27:115–28.
84. Ramirez S, McClure JJ, Moore RM, et al. Hyperthyroidism associated with a thyroid adenocarcinoma in a 21-year-old gelding. J Vet Intern Med 1998;12:475–7.

85. Alberts MK, McCann JP, Woods PR. Hemithyroidectomy in a horse with confirmed hyperthyroidism. J Am Vet Med Assoc 2000;217:1051–4.
86. Tan RH, Davies SE, Crisman MV, et al. Propylthiouracil for treatment of hyperthyroidism in a horse. J Vet Intern Med 2008;22:1253–8.
87. Peauroi JR, Fisher DJ, Mohr FC, et al. Primary hyperparathyroidism caused by a functional parathyroid adenoma in a horse. J Am Vet Med Assoc 1998;212: 1915–8.
88. Cottle HJ, Hughes KJ, Thompson H, et al. Primary hyperparathyroidism in a 17-year-old Arab × Welsh Cob pony mare with a functional parathyroid adenoma. Equine Vet Educ 2014. http://dx.doi.org/10.1111/eve.12183.
89. Wong D, Sponseller B, Miles K, et al. Failure of Technetium Tc 99m sestamibi scanning to detect abnormal parathyroid tissue in a horse and a mule with primary hyperparathyroidism. J Vet Intern Med 2004;18:589–93.
90. Tomlinson JE, Johnson AL, Ross MW, et al. Successful detection and removal of a functional parathyroid adenoma in a pony using technetium Tc 99m sestamibi scintigraphy. J Vet Intern Med 2014;28:687–92.
91. Barton MH, Sharma P, LeRoy BE, et al. Hypercalcemia and high serum parathyroid hormone-related protein concentration in a horse with multiple myeloma. J Am Vet Med Assoc 2004;225:409–13.
92. Taylor SD, Haldorson GJ, Vaughan B, et al. Gastric neoplasia in horses. J Vet Intern Med 2009;23:1097–102.
93. van der Kolk JH, Ijzer J, Overgaauw PA, et al. Pituitary-independent Cushing's syndrome in a horse. Equine Vet J 2001;33:110–2.
94. Germann SE, Rütten M, Derungs SB, et al. Multiple endocrine neoplasia-like syndrome in a horse. Vet Rec 2006;159:530–2.
95. Herbach N, Nagel L, Zwick T, et al. Multiple glucagon-producing pancreatic neuroendocrine tumors in a horse (Equus caballus). Vet Pathol 2014;51:607–11.
96. Johnson PJ, Goetz TE, Foreman JH, et al. Pheochromocytoma in two horses. J Am Vet Med Assoc 1995;206:837–41.

Exercise and Rehabilitation of Older Horses

Kenneth Harrington McKeever, MS, PhD

KEYWORDS

- Aging • Horse • Physiologic function • Exercise capacity

KEY POINTS

- The population of older horses is increasing, with many of those animals performing various athletic activities into their 20s.
- Published studies have focused on the physiologic mechanisms associated with the onset of aging-induced decreases in physiologic function and exercise capacity in the horse.
- The information presented can be used as a guide for exercise prescriptions for the growing population of athletically active older equine athletes.

INTRODUCTION

In 1996, researchers conducted the first study that compared the physiologic markers of exercise capacity in young mature and old horses.[1] The old horses were all more than 20 years of age and, as expected, there was a substantial difference in maximal aerobic capacity and the amount of anaerobic work that the old horses could perform compared with the young mature horses.[1] An unexpected observation was that there was no increase of muscle enzyme levels in both groups of horses, suggesting no detrimental effect of the intense exercise on the old horses.[1] Questions arose out of that experiment, regarding the benefits of moderate exercise training for older horses that are sound and healthy. Aging seems to alter metabolic control, immune function, and endocrine function in horses, both at rest and following exercise.[2,3] Older horses may undergo significant changes in body composition, with some horses losing muscle mass and some becoming obese.[4–6] There are many changes associated with aging that can limit the ability to perform light or moderate exercise and the question

Disclosure: This work was supported by funds from New Jersey Agricultural Experiment Station and the Rutgers Equine Science Center.
Department of Animal Science, Equine Science Center, School of Environmental and Biological Sciences, Rutgers, the State University of New Jersey, 84 Lipman Drive, New Brunswick, NJ 08901-8525, USA
E-mail address: mckeever@aesop.rutgers.edu

remains as to whether this is caused by inactivity or aging.[4–6] This article discusses how aging affects the systems important to any exercise activity, synthesizing information from exercise physiologists and veterinarians conducting basic and applied studies into a format that can serve as a guide for clinicians contemplating an exercise prescription for older horses.

AGE-RELATED CHANGES IN AEROBIC CAPACITY AND CARDIOVASCULAR FUNCTION

It is well known that, in humans, the ability to perform strenuous work decreases with age, both because of a decline in aerobic capacity and a decline in anaerobic power.[7,8] However, much debate exists in the literature as to how much of that decline is caused by physiologic aging versus disease process related to inactivity. Aging seems to have profound effects on the cardiovascular system, producing decreases in maximal heart rate (HR_{max}), changes in baroreceptor sensitivity, decreased vascular compliance, and hypertension in species such as rats, dogs, and humans.[9–11] These observations have led to a fine tuning of exercise prescription for older human athletes to prevent the adverse and potentially dangerous effects of excessive work.[7,12]

Both older humans and horses show a decline in maximal oxygen uptake (Vo_{2max}) and exercise capacity. McKeever and Malinowski[1] showed that submaximal oxygen consumption was similar in young and old horses subjected to an incremental exercise test. However, Vo_{2max}, was significantly lower in unfit horses more than 20 years old ($\sim$90 mL/kg/min) compared with unfit young horses less than 10 years old ($\sim$120 mL/kg/min). As expected, the amount of work needed to reach Vo_{2max} was lower in the older horses.[1] That study also suggested that there was a decline in the capacity to tolerate high-intensity exercise because older horses fatigued at lower exercise intensities than young animals.[1]

In terms of physiologic age the older horses in the study mentioned earlier were analogous to humans, ranging from 60 to 78 years of age, but horses' innate aerobic capacity is vastly greater than in humans. A study of moderately fit, healthy, postmenopausal women reported maximal aerobic capacities averaging 22 mL/kg/min.[2,7] Elite, Olympic-caliber, human athletes typically have maximal aerobic capacities in the 60 to 80 mL/kg/min.[13] Elite fit horses have maximal rates of oxygen consumption more than 145 mL/kg/min. The older mares in the experiment mentioned earlier with an average Vo_{2max} of 90 mL/kg/min were less than their fit equine counterparts, but still well above the levels reported for young, fit, elite human athletes.[1]

One benefit of having a greater aerobic capacity in younger horses was the delay in the need to increase the rate of anaerobic glycolysis to fuel higher intensity exercise.[1] Younger horses had to exercise harder before reaching the anaerobic threshold or the point where the onset of blood lactate accumulation is observed; a point marked by blood lactate concentration of $\sim$4 mMol/L.[1,3] At this point there is a curvilinear increase in blood lactate concentration indicative that lactate production by the working muscles has greatly exceeded lactate use throughout the rest of the body.[3] This variable is important because the velocity to produce a blood lactate concentration of 4 mMol/L (V_{LA4}) coincides with changes in several important physiologic processes related to regulation of acid-base status as well as respiration. It is also considered an indicator of endurance capacity. The older horses reached the V_{LA4} at both a lower speed and at a lower relative work intensity.[3]

Mechanistically, the decline in Vo_{2max} seems to be caused by central factors (heart) as well peripheral factors (muscle) that limit oxygen delivery and use.[14,15] This process can be better understood by examining the effects of aging on the components of the Fick equation, in which:

Formula 1: Vo_2 = Cardiac output $\times$ (a $-$ v)O_2

Formula 2: Cardiac output = Heart rate $\times$ Stroke volume

The (a $-$ v)O_2, or the difference between oxygen content measured in arterial and venous blood samples, represents the extraction or use of oxygen. Anything that alters one of the components of the Fick equation will affect the ability to deliver and use oxygen. Old mares (mean age 27 years) had a lower HR_{max} both before (193 $\pm$ 3 beats/min) and after training (198 $\pm$ 2 beats/min), although this decline was not seen in mares with a mean age of 15 years.[14] This aging-related decline in HR_{max} from ~228 beats/min in the young mature horses seems to be one factor that limits maximal cardiac output and, thus, maximal aerobic capacity (Vo_{2max}) in horses as well as humans.[7,14]

The effect of aging on HR_{max} is important because it affects the strategy for the use of heart rate monitoring and target heart rates to set the intensity of an exercise training program. In heart rate–based training programs for humans the training intensity is adjusted to produce a target heart rate between 50% and 85% of the age-predicted HR_{max}. The low target of 50% of age-predicted HR_{max}, represents the minimal work intensity needed to induce a beneficial cardiovascular adaptation. Work at more than 85% of HR_{max} involves increasingly greater contributions from anaerobic metabolic pathways. The decline in HR_{max} seen with aging means that horse owners need to reduce absolute exercise intensities to safely produce a training effect without compromising other physiologic systems. A large number of human studies were used to establish that the age-predicted HR_{max} can be calculated by subtracting the person's age from 220 beats/min. Similar research is limited in the horse to the single study by Vincent and colleagues,[16] which used data from the laboratories of several international collaborators (including Ref.[7]) to establish a regression equation for predicting HR_{max} in horses. Many factors affecting HR_{max}, such as fitness status, body weight, and breed, were found to alter the prediction of HR_{max}.[16] However, they suggested that for each year older than a baseline (2-year-old horse; 224 beats/min), HR_{max} decreased by 0.86 beats per minute. With all their variables at baseline, a 22-year-old horse would have an age-predicted HR_{max} 17 beats/min lower than a 2-year-old of similar breed, and so forth.[16] Follow-up studies are needed to establish a prediction equation that can be readily used for training older horses.

To better define when changes in cardiopulmonary function become apparent in horses as they age, Walker and colleagues [17] conducted a retrospective study of all the horses tested in their exercise physiology laboratory between 1995 and 2009. Ages of the horses ranged between 4 and 29 years.[17] The study documented that the decline in aerobic capacity started between 18 and 20 years (**Fig. 1**), although this breakpoint may vary depending on genetic influences, health status, and amount of prior training. Practically, when prescribing exercise for an older horse, baseline and past fitness levels as well as age are important, with exercise in older, unfit horses needing to be built up slowly and carefully.

Studies of humans have suggested that the decrease in HR_{max} with age results from several mechanisms, including aging-induced changes in the number of pacemaker cells in the sinoatrial node, increases in the elastic and collagenous tissue in all parts of the conduction system, and the deposition of adipose tissue around the sinoatrial node.[10,18] In humans, aging seems to also affect autonomic control of the heart,

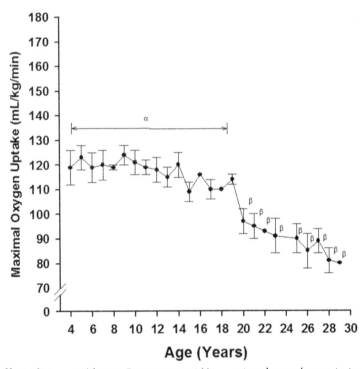

Fig. 1. Effect of Vo$_{2max}$ with age. Data represent Vo$_{2max}$ at each year (mean ± standard error). Values were obtained from graded exercise tests run on a sample size of 50 unfit standardbred mares. As the Vo$_{2max}$ drops gradually with age, there is a clear breakpoint between the ages of 18 and 20 years. Points marked α are statistically the same as age 4 years. Points marked β are statistically different than age 4 years. (*From* Walker A, Arent SM, McKeever KH. Maximal aerobic capacity (Vo$_{2MAX}$) in horses: a retrospective study to identify the age-related decline. Comp Exerc Physiol 2009;6:177–81; with permission.)

with a downregulation of the heart's sensitivity to the sympathetic nervous system reducing heart rate increases during exercise.[10]

Aging in the horse also seems to affect the heart itself as well as the autonomic control of heart rate, which may explain the major part of the decrease in central cardiovascular capacity in the horse. Betros and colleagues[19] showed that the intrinsic heart rate (the heart rate observed without the influence of autonomic nervous control) differed in young and old horses and that training-induced alterations in intrinsic heart rate only occurred in young horses. Indirect evidence suggests that the horse may also undergo aging-induced changes in the neuroendocrine control of heart rate and cardiovascular function during exercise.[20–22]

In addition, when considering the decline in aerobic capacity, the contribution of peripheral cardiovascular factors in the decline in exercise performance seen in horses, dogs, and humans cannot be ruled out.[10,14,18,19,23] Some of the decline in aerobic capacity may be caused by changes in peripheral mechanisms affecting the ability to use oxygen, including decreased muscle mass, alterations in muscle capillary density, and decreased vascular compliance, which may also limit exercise capacity by limiting blood flow to working muscles.[24,25] However, most of these data have been extrapolated from submaximal studies and the debate continues on whether age-related declines in cardiovascular capacity in humans are predominated by central or peripheral mechanisms.

AGE-RELATED CHANGES IN THERMOREGULATION AND FLUID AND ELECTROLYTE BALANCE

Studies of the thermoregulatory responses of older and younger men and women during exercise in the heat have shown conclusively that age influences thermoregulatory function during exercise.[26–28] The impact of this decline in the ability to dissipate heat during exercise is even more critical when exercise is performed in hot and humid conditions.[27] This age-related decrease in the ability to thermoregulate during exercise in humans is caused by an age-related decrease in cardiac output as well as changes in the control of skin blood flow, and a possible state of hypohydration in the elderly.[27]

To date, there has been limited research addressing the decline in the thermoregulatory response to exercise in old horses, but it seems that older horses also have lower total body water volume, plasma volume, and reserves of fluid for sweating and thermoregulation.[27,29] McKeever and colleagues[30] exercised young (mean age 8 years) and old horses (mean age 26 years) at the same submaximal absolute work intensity of 1625 W until they reached a core body temperature of 40°C. The old horses reached a core temperature of 40°C in almost half the time required by the younger mares, with older mares having substantially higher heart rates at 40°C compared with the young mares.[30] Both groups had similar heart rates and core temperatures by 10 minutes after exercise. Markers of hydration status indicated they also had similar relative declines in plasma volume, but the old horses had started off with a substantially lower absolute plasma volume than younger horses.[30] The result was a lower reserve of fluid to provide for cardiovascular and thermoregulatory stability. In a follow-up experiment, Betros and colleagues[19] showed that old horses do not increase their plasma volume with training like younger animals. This lack of a training-induced hypervolemia is seen in older humans and may be related to a disruption of the renin-angiotensin-aldosterone cascade.

Another aspect of cooling that is affected by aging is the increase in skin blood flow that is needed to properly liberate heat from the body. It has been shown in older humans that there are 2 factors that contribute to this age-related phenomenon. First, the lower plasma and blood volumes mean that cardiac output is inadequate to support maximal blood flow to the muscles as well as maximal skin blood flow. This condition leads to compromised ability to dissipate heat and defend against hyperthermia.[27] In addition, Ho and colleagues[29] showed that there is an age-related disruption of local neuroendocrine control of skin blood flow during exercise in humans. The inability to keep cool despite an increase in sweat rate in older horses would be consistent with an impairment of skin blood flow as observed in humans. Work is needed to determine whether aging affects skin blood flow during exercise in the horse.

During high work intensities, the rate of heat production of the horse can exceed basal levels by 40-fold to 60-fold.[31,32] If the excess metabolic heat generated during exercise is not dissipated, performance-affecting or even life-threatening increases in body temperature may develop.[32] The increased susceptibility of older horses to overheating should be considered by veterinarians, owners, and riders and the appropriate precautions should be taken to prevent exercise-induced hyperthermia in older horses during equine athletic events. Firstly, the environmental conditions need to be monitored and riding or competition should be avoided when it is hot and humid. Secondly, owners should be aware of the hydration status of their horses and provide opportunities to drink.[33] Assessments should be performed of temperature, pulse, and respiration when possible, or owners should be keenly aware of what is normal for their exercising older horses. Note that the adverse effects of hyperthermia on the health and performance of horses can develop during all exercise intensities and weather conditions, but these recommendations are especially critical for horses that are not adapted to exercise in the heat.

AGING-INDUCED CHANGES IN RESPIRATORY FUNCTION THAT MAY AFFECT EXERCISE

Factors affecting lung health can have a cumulative effect in the horse and ultimately cause a decrement in respiratory function during exertion.[34] Over a lifetime older horses can be exposed to more pathogens and allergens, which can lead to an increased prevalence of small airway disease and recurrent airway obstruction.[34] Although research in horses is sparse, in humans aging has been shown to have a significant effect on lung function during exercise.[18] A review by Dempsey and Seals[18] suggests that there are several aging-related alterations in pulmonary function that limit respiratory capacity in older humans, including an expiratory flow limitation at lower work intensities and a decrease in the end-expiratory lung volume suggested to be caused by altered elastic recoil of the lung.[18] Older individuals also seem to have a greater dead space, which affects the dead space/tidal volume ratio.[18] They also report that in older humans the work of breathing is increased during exertion and that lung hemodynamics are affected by aging-induced decreases in arteriolar compliance, which in turn may lead to capillary stress failure.[18] Capillary stress failure may have implications for the horse because it is part of the cause of exercise-induced pulmonary hemorrhage.[18] Despite all of these age-related changes in lung physiology, alveolar to arterial gas exchange and pulmonary vascular hemodynamics are only slightly modified by aging in humans.[18] It would be interesting to determine whether similar patterns of aging-induced changes in lung function seen in humans are present in old horses.[34]

EFFECTS OF AGE ON BODY COMPOSITION AND MUSCLE FIBER TYPE

Another measure that may have an important bearing on the ability to perform exercise is body composition and, more importantly, total fat-free mass (FFM).[35] The predominant component of a horse's FFM is muscle mass and a strong correlation between FFM and performance has been documented in elite standardbred horses.[35] Older humans show substantial decreases in muscle mass and in many cases increases in fat mass that affect the ability to perform exercise.[8,36–40] However, Malinowski and colleagues[6] reported no differences between unfit old (mean age 8 years), middle-aged (mean age 15 years), and young (mean age 27 years) mares for total body weight, rump fat thickness, percentage body fat, or fat weight before training. A later study found significant age-related differences in pretraining body composition when the horses were separated by morphometric appearance.[5] It was reported that the old horses (mean age ±20 years) could be divided into 2 groups, with some horses that were either very lean or very fat.[5] The very lean old mares had significantly smaller rump fat thickness, lower percentage body fat, and less fat weight than both the fat old mares and the young mares (4–8 years).[5] In turn, the old fat group had a significantly larger rump fat thickness, percentage body fat, and fat weight compared with the young mares.[5]

Exercise training has a beneficial effect on body composition in older horses.[4,6] Malinowski and colleagues[6] reported that after 12 weeks of training old horses (±20 years) had an 8% increase in FFM (ie, muscle mass) and a highly significant 24% decrease in fat mass. In a later study, Aulisio and colleagues[4] measured body composition after 8 and 15 weeks of training in young (mean age 7 years) and old (mean age 22 years) horses and found that there was a nonsignificant progressive decrease in fat mass and a significant increase in FFM that became significant only after 15 weeks of submaximal exercise training. The velocity and duration of exercise were increased gradually over the course of both experiments to prevent exercise-associated injuries in the horses.

Although old horses seem to retain muscle mass, it is important to ask whether that is functional muscle mass? That question can only be addressed by studying muscle fiber profiles, enzyme concentrations, and substrate concentrations. Few studies have examined peripheral changes associated with aging in the horse and those studies have focused on changes in fiber type associated with aging.[5,41,42] Riviero and colleagues[41] examined muscle fiber type distribution in several horses and found that there were age-related differences. However, the mean age of the oldest age group in that study was only 15 years, an age at which many horses are still in their prime athletically and physiologically; analogous to humans aged 40 years or more.[41] Another study compared young and old horses (20–29 years) and found that aged mares had fewer type I and IIA fibers and more type IIX fibers than the young mature horses.[5] On a functional level the investigators suggested that the older horses had a switch in fiber type population away from the type that would be favorable to endurance exercise. It was further suggested that those observations may, in part, explain the decrease in maximal aerobic capacity documented in other studies.[1,17] The documented change in muscle fiber profile is similar to the change observed in disuse atrophy models such as hind limb suspension in rats and space flight models in humans, Rhesus monkeys, and rats.[43–55]

On a cellular level, aging seems to significantly alter muscle structure and function in species other than horses.[43–52,54,55] Studies in rats and humans show that connective tissue content in the muscle is altered with increased amounts of collagen.[8,16] These changes interfere with normal contractile function. Other studies have reported conflicting results regarding skeletal muscle blood capillarity in aged humans, some indicating no change with age and some showing a significant age-related decline.[25] However, blood flow has been reported to be lower in older men.[23,56] Oxidative capacity also declines with age in old humans and other animals.[46,47,57] Glucose use seems to be reduced in older humans, possibly through changes in GLUT-4 activity and insulin insensitivity.[28,44,56,58] In addition, glycogen depletion/repletion patterns in skeletal muscle seem to be altered by age in rats and humans.[25,44,45,59] However, no data have been published for the effect of exercise on muscle enzyme concentrations or glycogen depletion and repletion patterns in old horses. Age-induced alterations in those metabolic control mechanisms may be important because they would affect the ability both to exercise and to recover from exercise.

AGING-RELATED ALTERATIONS IN THE ENDOCRINE RESPONSE TO EXERCISE

Exercise involves the integration of multiple organ systems that communicate via neural and endocrine pathways. Humans undergo substantial alterations in neural control mechanisms, with primary alterations in sympathetic nervous system responsiveness.[2,24,39,57,60] No such information exists for the horse. Aging also alters the endocrine response to exercise with reported changes in hormone levels associated with the control of cardiovascular function, stress hormones, and endocrine/paracrine factors related to the control of metabolic function and substrate use.[2,24,39,57,60]

Cardiovascular and Renal Hormones

Alterations in the renin-angiotensin-aldosterone (RAA) cascade with age may be physiologically important because it is a well-recognized part of the acute defense of blood pressure during exercise as well as the long-term control of fluid and electrolyte balance after exercise. More specifically, circulating angiotensin I and II aid in the vasoconstriction that occurs in nonobligate tissues that is part of the redistribution of blood flow.[61,62] Angiotensin also stimulates thirst and causes an increase in the synthesis and release of aldosterone. McKeever and Malinowski[63] observed age-related differences in the RAA cascade in old horses, similar to observations reported for healthy old humans and other species.[27,62] They found similar resting concentrations of atrial natriuretic peptide (ANP), arginine vasopressin, plasma renin activity (PRA), aldosterone, and endothelin-1 (ET-1) in healthy old and young horses.[63,64] Old and young horses had directionally similar exercise-induced alterations in PRA, ANP, vasopressin, and aldosterone, but there was an aging-related change in the magnitude of the response to exertion, reflecting differences in sensitivity in the regulation of blood pressure and blood flow during exertion.[63] Although old horses had different concentrations of these hormones, the observed concentrations were still within the range of normal for maximally exercised horses and other species.[27,61,62] The young horses had a greater increase in levels of the vasodilator ANP, which inhibits PRA and also inhibits the production and release of antagonistic hormones like vasopressin, and aldosterone. In contrast, older horses had greater PRA at speeds eliciting Vo_{2max}.[63] Functionally, greater concentrations of plasma ANP in younger animals enhance the ability to optimally vasodilate blood vessels in the periphery, especially in the working muscles.[61,62]

Surprisingly, younger horses seem to have a greater vasopressin response during acute exercise.[63] Vasopressin functions independently of the RAA system in the defense of blood volume and blood pressure during exercise. Plasma vasopressin concentration increases when the cardiopulmonary baroreceptors sense that cardiac filling pressure is inadequate, when the high-pressure baroreceptors sense that mean arterial blood pressure is too low, and/or when hypothalamic osmoreceptors sense that plasma osmolality is too high.[61,62] Vasopressin causes vasoconstriction in nonobligate tissues during exercise. It also facilitates the uptake of water and electrolytes from the large intestine, which is another important action during exercise.[61,62] After exercise, vasopressin causes a retention of solute-free water by the kidney and stimulates thirst and drinking.[61,62] Some studies suggest that aged humans do not drink as much and many times are hypohydrated.[27,65] Suppression of thirst and drinking is an important consideration for those concerned with postevent care of older horses.

Age-related changes in baroreceptor sensitivity as well differences in autonomic control and input from the sympathetic nervous system alter renal sympathetic nerve activity and the stimulation of the juxtaglomerular apparatus.[27,66] This alteration affects the response of the RAA cascade to acute exertion and may play a role in the decline of the adaptive response to training and the failure of training to increase plasma and blood volume in older horses.[30]

Growth Hormone

It is well recognized that older horses have lower plasma concentrations of the thyroid hormones, somatotropin, and insulinlike growth factor-I compared with young animals, suggesting an age-related decline in the somatotropic axis in horses that is similar to that observed in other mammalian species.[67–69] Decreased somatotropin level is associated with many aging-induced changes, including decreases in cardio-pulmonary function, decreased aerobic exercise capacity, decreased immune function, impaired nutrient use, decreased nitrogen retention, and decreased lean body mass.[67,68] Similar changes have been observed in other species and there are comparative physiologic data from rats, dogs, and humans that have shown that there is a causal relationship between plasma concentrations of somatotropin and what has been termed the aging phenotype.[8,25]

Endorphin and Cortisol: the Stress Hormones

Endorphins and cortisol have been used as markers of the degree of physiologic stress during exercise.[70,71] The release of these hormones is a normal response to exercise, linked to duration and intensity of exercise, and their release may provide protection from the physiologic challenge of exertion.[70,71] Beta-endorphin functions as a natural opiate, forestalling the central mechanisms that would induce fatigue.[70,71] Cortisol functions as a metabolic hormone during exercise, influencing glucose metabolism.[70,71] After exercise, cortisol exerts a degree of antiinflammatory and immunosuppressive activity, possibly aiding in the repair of tissue altered by exertion and protecting against the inflammation associated with overexertion.

The effects of age and training on the release of beta-endorphin have been studied in horses.[70] Before training, beta-endorphin level increased by 5 minutes following exercise in all mares.[70] After training, beta-endorphin level was higher compared with before training in all 3 age groups; however, the peak in the old mares occurred later and was lower than in the other groups.[70] In that same study the investigators reported that cortisol levels increased by 5 minutes postexercise in young and middle-aged mares before and after training.[70] There was no exercise-induced increase in cortisol concentration either before or after training in old mares. The investigators interpreted this as an inappropriately low response to exercise and suggested that aging may have altered the hypothalamic-pituitary-adrenal axis (HPAA).

A follow-up study by Liburt and colleagues[72] used a series of endocrine stimulation tests to determine mechanistically how aging disrupts the HPAA. Training improved the sensitivity of the pituitary gland to corticotropin-releasing factor in both old and young mares (Liburt NR, Smarsh D, Avenatti R, et al. Response of the equine HPA axis to acute, intense exercise before and after training in old vs young standardbred mares. Submitted for publication).[72,73] However, the investigators also observed that the pituitary was not as sensitive to negative feedback from cortisol in older mares (Liburt NR, Smarsh D, Avenatti R, et al. Response of the equine HPA axis to acute, intense exercise before and after training in old vs young standardbred mares. Submitted for publication).[72,73] They suggested that chronic training exercise promoted a longer increase of adrenocorticotropic hormone (ACTH) level and an increase in adrenal activity (Liburt NR, Smarsh D, Avenatti R, et al. Response of the equine HPA axis to acute, intense exercise before and after training in old vs young standardbred mares. Submitted for publication). The investigators concluded that older animals can improve HPAA function by maintaining a moderate amount of physical activity and that training seemed to sensitize the adrenal glands of young mares to ACTH to a greater degree than old mares.

Metabolic Hormones and the Control of Glucose Homeostasis

Aging is frequently associated with glucose intolerance and insulin resistance in both humans and horses and regular exercise activity elicits several favorable responses that contribute to healthy aging.[74–78] In a study on the effects of aging and training on the glucose and insulin response following acute exertion in horses, old horses required greater concentrations of insulin to successfully manage their response to an oral glucose tolerance test.[6] Twelve weeks of exercise training resulted in a post–graded exercise test increase in insulin in all age groups.[6] Exercise training altered the insulin and glucose response to acute exercise more in the old horses, which was interpreted to suggest an improvement in insulin sensitivity in the older animals. Liburt and colleagues[73] conducted a follow-up study and reported that exercise training increased muscle mass and improved insulin sensitivity in geriatric and young mature horses.[73] However, in their old horses training did not completely restore insulin sensitivity to the level observed in young mares.[73] Proposed mechanisms for the positive effects of exercise include reduction in liver and muscle glycogen, increased binding of insulin to the insulin receptor and increased glucose uptake by muscle cell glucose transporters.[79] To that end, Avenatti and colleagues (Avenatti RC, McKeever KH, Horohov DW, et al. Malinowski HSP70 and HSP90 gene expression and protein content in whole blood and skeletal muscle in female standardbred horses. Submitted for publication) showed that aging alters the response of heat shock proteins and other signaling proteins to acute submaximal exercise and thus may explain some of the differences in the handling of glucose in old and young horses (Avenatti RC, McKeever KH, Horohov DW, et al. Malinowski effects of age and submaximal exercise on physiological markers of stress and inflammatory cytokines in standardbred mares. Submitted for publication).

ALTERATIONS IN THE IMMUNE RESPONSE TO EXERCISE

Studies of humans have shown that aging alters the immune response in general and, more importantly, the immune response to the challenge of exercise.[80,81] Similarly in older horses there seems to be an effect of aging on the immune response to acute exertion.[70,82] Horohov and colleagues[82] reported that there were differences in the immune systems of young (mean age 7.5 years) and old (mean age 25 years) horses both before and after exertion. Old horses showed lower mononuclear cell proliferative responses to mitogens, suggesting an aging-related alteration in T cell–mediated function and an immunosenescence.[82] Acute exercise caused a decrease in the lymphoproliferation response in the younger horses but not the old mares.[82] The investigators suggested that the concurrent finding of a lower cortisol response to exertion in the old horses compared with young horses may explain the differences in the immune responses between the groups.[82] In contrast, the mitogen-stimulated lymphoproliferative response following simulated race tests both before and after training was reduced in old compared with young and middle-aged mares in another study.[70] That study also measured the immune responses to a graded exercise test performed before and after 12 weeks' training at 60% of HR_{max} in young, middle aged, and old mares.[70] The investigators measured leukocyte cell number, CD4+ and CD8+ cell subsets, and the lymphoproliferative response to mitogenic challenge and found significant age and training effects.[70] The older horses had lower monocyte counts after graded exercise test after training.[5] Lymphocyte numbers increased in all mares after exercise, with age having an effect as shown by different levels in the middle-aged and old mares.[70] Note that the CD4+ lymphocyte counts were higher at rest in old and middle-aged mares compared with younger mares.[70] Furthermore, age had a profound effect with a reduction in CD4+ lymphocyte levels seen in the old and middle-aged but not the young horses following the pre-training graded exercise test.[70] It was also stated that age had no effect on resting CD8+ lymphocytes and that training resulted in an increase in all groups.[5] These studies support the contention that extra attention to preventive health care (eg, vaccination) may be needed for older athletic horses.

RENAL, GASTROINTESTINAL, AND OTHER SYSTEMS

Research using humans has suggested that many of the observed changes in renal function seen with aging are inevitable and are the combined effect of disorders coupled with the aging process. There are limited data on the effect of age on the renal response to acute exercise in humans.[27,66] Those studies have primarily focused on the effect of aging on the normal reduction in blood flow seen with acute exertion.[27,66] Functionally older individuals have smaller reductions in renal blood flow and smaller increases in skin blood flow compared with younger humans.[27,66] This difference may alter renal function as well as thermoregulatory capacity because the redistribution of blood flow away from nonobligate tissues toward the working muscles and skin are important responses to exertion.[27,66] No work has been performed in the horse; however, a reduction in skin blood flow would alter the ability to thermoregulate and may explain some of the differences in thermoregulatory capacity reported in older horses. Aging-induced alterations in renal sympathetic nerve activity and the RAA cascade may play a role in the change in blood flow distribution in humans.[27,66] This hypothesized mechanism may play a role in the horse because it is the only species other than humans that sweats to thermoregulate during exercise and, as mentioned, older horses have an altered PRA response to exertion.[63] More work is also needed to determine whether aging alters mechanisms affecting the glomerular filtration rate and tubular function both during exercise and afterward, which may be important because long-term control of total body water, plasma volume, and fluid and electrolyte balance seem to be altered in humans and horses.

Other systems altered with age in other species include the gastrointestinal tract and bones and ligaments as well as the integumentary system.[2] Changes in the gastrointestinal tract from dental wear to decreased absorptive capability all influence the uptake of water and nutrients and have the potential to alter the ability to perform exercise.[83–85] Bone disorder ranging from osteoarthritis to demineralization can alter the ability to perform exercise in old horses. Changes in the skin have the potential to alter sweating and thermoregulation. However, the authors are unaware of any data on the effects of age on these systems in the horse.

SUMMARY

Surveys indicate that up to 15% of the equine population in the United States is more than 20 years of age, with many of those animals performing various athletic activities well into their 20s.[3,86,87] Despite clear advantages of exercise on health and physiology for all ages, exercise training protocols that are appropriate for younger animals may not be appropriate for older horses.[13,24,27,88,89] Studies of aged humans have led to a fine tuning of exercise prescription for older human athletes to prevent the adverse and potential dangerous effects of excessive exercise.[52,56] Published results have led to new and improved programs to promote fitness for the growing population of older adult humans. More studies of the effects of aging on exercise capacity in equine athletes are needed to address the age at which physiologic function first begins to decline and to determine what levels of exercise will enhance the health and well-being of older horses without harm.

REFERENCES

1. McKeever KH, Malinowski K. Exercise capacity in young and old female horses. Am J Vet Res 1997;58:1468–72.
2. Holloszy JO, Kohrt WM. Exercise. In: Masoro EJ, editor. Handbook of physiology, section 11, aging. New York: Oxford University Press; 1995. p. 633–66. Chapter 24.
3. McKeever KH. Exercise physiology of the older horse. In: MacLeay JM, editor. Veterinary clinics of North America: equine practice; geriatrics, vol. 18. Philadelphia: Saunders; 2002. p. 469–90.
4. Aulisio JL, Libut NR, Malinowski K, et al. Training-induced alterations in rump fat thickness and plasma leptin concentration in young and old Standardbred mares. Comp Exerc Physiol 2011;7:127–32.
5. Lehnhard RA, McKeever KH, Kearns CF, et al. Myosin heavy chain profiles and body composition are different in old versus young Standardbred mares. The Vet J 2004;167:59–66.
6. Malinowski K, Betros CL, Flora L, et al. Effect of training on age-related changes in plasma insulin and glucose. Equine Vet J Suppl 2002;34:147–53.
7. Raven PB, Mitchell JH. Effect of aging on the cardiovascular response to dynamic and static exercise. In: Westfeldt ML, editor. The aging heart: its function and response to stress. New York: Raven Press; 1980. p. 269–96.
8. Stamford BA. Exercise and the elderly. In: Pandolf KB, editor. Exercise and Sport science reviews, vol. 16. New York: MacMillan Publishing Company; 1988. p. 341–80.
9. Hornig B, Maier V, Drexler H. Physical training improves endothelial function in patients with chronic heart failure. Circulation 1996;93:210–4.
10. Lakatta EG. Cardiovascular System. In: Masoro EJ, editor. Handbook of physiology, section 11, aging. New York: Oxford University Press; 1995. p. 413–74. Chapter 17.
11. Predel HG, Meyer-Lehnert H, Backer A, et al. Plasma concentrations of endothelin in patients with abnormal vascular reactivity: effects of ergometric exercise and acute saline loading. Life Sci 1990;47:1837–43.
12. Ready AE, Naimark B, Ducas J, et al. Influence of walking volume on health benefits in women post-menopause. Med Sci Sports Exer 1996;28:1097–105.
13. Haskell WL, Phillips WT. Exercise training, fitness, health, and longevity. In: Lamb DR, Gisolfi CV, Nadel E, editors. Perspectives in exercise and sports medicine, Exercise in older adults, vol. 8. Carmel (IN): Cooper Publishing; 1995. p. 11–52.
14. Betros CL, McKeever KH, Kearns CF, et al. Effects of ageing and training on maximal heart rate and VO_{2max}. Equine Vet J Suppl 2002;34:100–5.
15. Haidet GC, Parsons D. Reduced exercise capacity in senescent beagles: an evaluation of the periphery. Am J Physiol 1991;260:H173–82.
16. Vincent TL, Newton JR, Deaton CM, et al. A retrospective study of predictive variables for maximal heart rate in horses undergoing strenuous treadmill exercise. Equine Vet J Suppl 2006;36:146–52.
17. Walker A, Arent SM, McKeever KH. Maximal aerobic capacity (VO_{2MAX}) in horses: a retrospective study to identify the age-related decline. Comp Exerc Physiol 2009;6:177–81.
18. Dempsey JA, Seals DR. Aging, exercise, and cardiopulmonary function. In: Lamb DR, Gisolfi CV, Nadel E, editors. Perspectives in exercise and sports

medicine, Exercise in older adults, vol. 8. Carmel (IN): Cooper Publishing; 1995. p. 237–304.

19. Betros CL, McKeever NM, Malinowski K, et al. Effects of aging and training on resting and intrinsic heart rate in horses. Comp Exerc Physiol 2013;9:43–50.

20. Goetz TE, Manohar M. Isoproterenol-induced maximal heart rate in normothermic and hyperthermic horses. Am J Vet Res 1990;51:743–6.

21. Gunn HM. Relative increase in areas of muscle fibre types in horses during growth. Equine Vet J Suppl 1995;18:209–13.

22. Guy PS, Snow DH. The Effect of training and detraining on muscle composition in the horse. J Physiol 1977;269(1):33–51.

23. Meridith CN, Frontera WR, Fisher EC, et al. Peripheral effects of endurance training in young and old subjects. J Appl Physiol 1989;66:2844–9.

24. Seals DR. Influence of aging on autonomic-circulatory control at rest and during exercise in humans. In: Gisolfi CV, Lamb DR, Nadel E, editors. Perspectives in exercise science and sports medicine, Exercise, heat, and thermoregulation, vol. 6. Dubuque (IA): WC Brown; 1993. p. 257–97.

25. White T. Skeletal muscle structure and function in older mammals. In: Lamb DR, Gisolfi CV, Nadel E, editors. In: Lamb DR, Gisolfi CV, Nadel E, editors. Perspectives in exercise and sports medicine, Exercise in older adults, vol. 8. Carmel, IN: Cooper Publishing; 1995. p. 115–74.

26. Armstrong CG, Kenney WL. Effects of age and acclimation on responses to passive heat exposure. J Appl Physiol 1993;75:2162–7.

27. Kenney WL. Body fluid and temperature regulation as a function of age. In: Lamb DR, Gisolfi CV, Nadel E, editors. Perspectives in exercise and sports medicine, Exercise in older adults, vol. 8. Carmel (IN): Cooper Publishing; 1995. p. 305–51.

28. Tankersley CG, Smolander J, Kenney WL, et al. Sweating and skin blood flow during exercise: effects of age and maximal oxygen uptake. J Appl Physiol 1991;71: 236–42.

29. Ho CW, Beard JL, Farrell PA, et al. Age, fitness, and regional blood flow during exercise in the heat. J Appl Physiol 1997;82:1126–35.

30. McKeever KH, Eaton TL, Geiser S, et al. Aging related decreases in thermoregulation and cardiovascular function. Equine Vet J 2010;42(S38):220–7.

31. Geor RJ, McCutcheon LJ, Ecker Gayle L, et al. Thermal and cardiorespiratory responses of horses to submaximal exercise under hot and humid conditions. Equine Vet J Suppl 1995;20:125–32.

32. McConaghy F. Thermoregulation. In: Hodgson DR, Rose RJ, editors. The athletic horse: principles and practice of equine sports medicine. Philadelphia: Saunders; 1994. p. 181–91.

33. Naylor JR, Bayly WM, Gollnick PD, et al. Effects of dehydration on thermoregulatory responses of horses during low-intensity exercise. J Appl Physiol 1993;75: 994–1000.

34. Lekeux P, Art T. The respiratory system: anatomy, physiology, and adaptations to exercise and training. In: Hodgson DR, Rose RJ, editors. The athletic horse: principles and practice of equine sports medicine. Philadelphia: Saunders; 1994. p. 79–128.

35. Kearns CF, McKeever KH, Abe T. Overview of horse body composition and muscle architecture- implications for performance. Vet J 2002;64:224–34.

36. Forbes GB, Reina JC. Adult lean body mass declines with age: some longitudinal observations. Metab Clin Exp 1970;19:653–63.

37. Freestone JF, Shoemaker K, Bessin R, et al. Insulin and glucose response following oral glucose administration in well-conditioned ponies. Equine Vet J Suppl 1992;11:13–7.

38. Frontera WR, Hughes VA, Fielding RA, et al. Aging of skeletal muscle: a 12-yr longitudinal study. J Appl Physiol 2000;88:1321–6.

39. Kohrt WM, Spina RJ, Ehsani AA, et al. Effects of age, adiposity, and fitness level on plasma catecholamine responses to standing and exercise. J Appl Physiol 1993;75:1828–35.

40. Kohrt WM, Malley MT, Dalsky GP, et al. Body composition of healthy sedentary and trained, young and older men and women. Med Sci Sports Exerc 1992;24: 832–83.

41. Rivero JLL, Galisteo AM, Aguer E, et al. Skeletal muscle histochemistry in male and female Andalusian and Arabian horses of different ages. Res Vet Sci 1993; 54:160–9.

42. Roneus M, Lindholm A. Muscle characteristics in Thoroughbreds of different ages and sexes. Equine Vet J 1991;23:207–10.

43. Andersen JL, Terzis G, Kryger A. Increase in the degree of coexpression of myosin heavy chain isoforms in skeletal muscle fibers of the very old. Muscle Nerve 1999;22:449–54.

44. Cartee GD. Influence of age on skeletal muscle glucose transport and glycogen metabolism. Med Sci Sports Exerc 1994;26:577–85.

45. Cartee GD, Farrar RP. Exercise training induces glycogen sparing during exercise by old rats. J Appl Physiol 1988;64:259–65.

46. Coggan AR, Abduljalil AM, Swanson SC, et al. Muscle metabolism during exercise in young and older trained and endurance trained men. J Appl Physiol 1993;75:2125–33.

47. Coggan AR, Spina RJ, King DJ, et al. Histochemical and enzymatic characteristics of the gastrocnemius muscle of young and elderly men and women. J Gerontol 1992;47:B71–6.

48. Davies CTM, Thomas DO, White MJ. Mechanical properties of young and elderly muscle. Acta Med Scand Suppl 1988;711:219–26.

49. Desplanches D, Mayet MH, Sempore B, et al. Structural and functional responses to prolonged hindlimb suspension in rat muscle. J Appl Physiol 1987;63:558–63.

50. Eddinger TJ, Moss RL, Cassens RG. Fiber number and type composition in extensor digitorum longus, soleus, and diaphragm muscles with aging in Fisher 344 rats. J Histochem Cytochem 1985;33:1033–41.

51. Edgerton VR, Zhou MY, Ohira Y, et al. Human fiber size and enzymatic properties after 5 and 11 days of spaceflight. J Appl Physiol 1995;78:1733–9.

52. Ekelund LG, Haskell WL, Johnson JL, et al. Physical fitness in the prevention of cardiovascular mortality in asymptomatic North American men. New Engl J Med 1988;319:1379–84.

53. Essen-Gustavsson B, Lindholm A. Muscle Fibre characteristics of active and inactive Standardbred horses. Equine Vet J Suppl 1985;17:434–8.

54. Haida N, Fowler WM Jr, Abresch RT, et al. Effect of hind-limb suspension on young and adult skeletal muscle. I. Normal mice. Exp Neurol 1989;103:68–76.

55. Riley DA. Review of primary spaceflight-induced and secondary reloading-induced changes in slow antigravity muscles of rats. Adv Space Res 1998;21: 1073–5.

56. Holloszy JO. Exercise, health, and aging: a need for more information. Med Sci Sports Exerc 1993;15:1–5.

57. Rubany GM, Shepherd JT. Hypothetical role of endothelin in the control of the cardiovascular system. In: Rubanyi GM, editor. Endothelin. New York: Oxford University Press; 1992. p. 258–71.

58. Terada S, Yokozeki T, Kawanaka K, et al. Effects of high-intensity swimming training on GLUT-4 and glucose transport activity in rat skeletal muscle. J Appl Physiol 2001;90:2019–24.

59. Kurokawa T, Ozaki N, Sato E, et al. Rapid decrease of glycogen concentration in the hearts of senescence-accelerated mice during aging. Mech Aging Dev 1997; 97:227–36.

60. Hoffman BB, Chang H, Farahbakhsh ZT, et al. Age-related decrement in hormone-stimulated lipolysis. Am J Physiol 1994;247:E772–7.

61. McKeever KH, Hinchcliff KW. Neuroendocrine control of blood volume, blood pressure, and cardiovascular function in horses. Equine Vet J Suppl 1995;18: 77–81.

62. Wade CE, Freund BJ, Claybaugh JR. Fluid and electrolyte homeostasis during and following exercise: hormonal and non-hormonal factors. In: Claybaugh JR, Wade CE, editors. Hormonal regulation of fluid and electrolytes. New York: Plenum; 1989. p. 1–44.

63. McKeever KH, Malinowski K. Endocrine response to exercise in young and old horses. Equine Vet J Suppl 1999;30:561–6.

64. McKeever KH, Kearns CF, Antas LA. Endothelin response during and after exercise in horses. The Vet J 2002;164:41–9.

65. Maeda S, Miyauchi T, Waku T, et al. Plasma endothelin-1 level in athletes after exercise in a hot environment: exercise-induced dehydration contributes to increases in plasma endothelin-1. Life Sci 1996;58:1259–68.

66. Kenney WL, Zappe DH. Effect of age on renal blood flow during exercise. Aging (Milano) 1994;6:293–302.

67. Malinowski K, Christensen RA, Konopka A, et al. Feed intake, body weight, body condition score, musculation, and immunocompetence in aged mares given equine somatotropin. J Anim Sci 1997;75:2727–33.

68. Malinowski K, Christensen RA, Hafs HD, et al. Age and breed differences in thyroid hormones, insulin-like growth factor-I and IGF binding proteins in horses. J Anim Sci 1996;74:1936–42.

69. McKeever KH, Malinowski K, Christensen R, et al. Chronic equine somatotropin administration does not affect aerobic capacity or indices of exercise performance in geriatric horses. The Vet J 1998;155:19–25.

70. Malinowski K, Shock EM, Roegner V, et al. Plasma β-endorphin, cortisol, and immune responses to acute exercise are altered by age and exercise training in horses. Equine Vet J Suppl 2006;36:2267–73.

71. Mehl ML, Schott HC, Sarkar DK, et al. Effects of exercise intensity on plasma β-endorphin concentrations in horses. Am J Vet Res 2000;61:969–73.

72. Liburt NR, McKeever K, Smarsh D, et al. The hypothalamic-pituitary-adrenal axis response to stimulation tests before and after exercise training in old vs. young standardbred mares. J Anim Sci 2013;91:5208–19.

73. Liburt NR, Fugaro MN, Wunderlich EK, et al. The effect of age and exercise training on insulin sensitivity, fat and muscle tissue cytokine profiles and body composition of old and young Standardbred mares. Comp Exerc Physiol 2012; 8:173–87.

74. Lonnqvist F, Nyberg H, Wahrenberg H, et al. Catecholamine-induced lipolysis in adipose tissue of the elderly. J Clin Invest 1990;85:1614–21.

75. Reaven GM. Insulin resistance and aging: modulation by obesity and physical activity. In: Lamb DR, Gisolfi CV, Nadel E, editors. Perspectives in exercise and sports medicine, Exercise in older adults, vol. 8. Carmel, IN: Cooper Publishing; 1995. p. 395–428.

76. Sial S, Coggan AR, Carroll R, et al. Fat and carbohydrate metabolism during exercise in elderly and young subjects. Am J Physiol 1996;271:E983–9.

77. Snow DH, Billeter R, Jenny E. Myosin Types in equine skeletal muscle fibres. Res Vet Sci 1981;30:381–2.

78. Snow DH, Guy PS. Muscle fibre type composition of a number of limb muscles in different types of horses. Res Vet Sci 1980;28:137–44.

79. Firshman AM, Valberg SJ. Factors affecting clinical assessment of insulin sensitivity in horses. Equine Vet J 2007;39:567–75.

80. Fiatarone MA, Morley JE, Bloom ET, et al. The effect of exercise on natural killer cell activity in young and old subjects. J Gerontol 1989;44:M37–45.

81. Nieman DC. Immune function. In: Lamb DR, Gisolfi CV, Nadel E, editors. Perspectives in exercise and sports medicine, Exercise in older adults, vol. 8. Carmel (IN): Cooper Publishing; 1995. p. 435–61.

82. Horohov DW, Dimock AN, Gurinalda PD, et al. Effects of exercise on the immune response of young and old horses. Am J Vet Res 1999;60:643–7.

83. Ralston SL, Breuer LH. Field evaluation of a feed formulated for geriatric horses. J Equine Vet Sci 1996;16:334–8.

84. Ralston SL, Nockels CF, Squires EL. Differences in diagnostic test results and hematologic data between aged and young horses. Am J Vet Res 1988;49:1387–92.

85. Ralston SL. Effect of soluble carbohydrate content of pelleted diets on post prandial glucose and insulin profiles in horses. Pferdeheilkunde 1992;112–5.

86. Hintz HF. Nutrition of the geriatric horse. In: Proceedings cornell nutrition conference. Cornell University; 1995. p. 195–8.

87. Rich GA. Nutritional and managerial considerations of the aged equine. In: Proceedings of advanced equine management short course. Colorado State University; 1989. p. 121–3.

88. Seals DR, Reiling MJ. Effect of regular exercise on 24-hour arterial blood pressure in older hypertensive humans. Hypertension 1991;18:583–92.

89. Seals DR, Hagberg JM, Hurley BF, et al. Endurance training in older men and women: I. Cardiovascular responses to exercise. J Appl Physiol 1984;57:1024–9.

Immune Dysfunction in Aged Horses

Dianne McFarlane, DVM, PhD

KEYWORDS

- Immunosenescence • Adaptive immunity • Proinflammatory • Geriatric horse

KEY POINTS

- Aging in horses, as in people, is associated with changes in both adaptive and innate immune responses.
- Age-related progressive impairment in the ability to respond to pathogen challenge and an increased inflammatory reactivity may predispose the geriatric horse to many diseases of old age.
- The high prevalence of pituitary pars intermedia dysfunction (combined with the difficulty in establishing an early diagnosis) means that all aged horses should be considered at high risk of poor immune function and treated accordingly.
- More work is needed to better understand the interactions of age on immunity, vaccine response, and disease risk in the horse.

IMMUNOSENESCENCE

Immunosenescence is the term that describes age-associated remodeling of the immune system that occurs in the elderly, resulting in poor immunity and an exaggerated inflammatory state. In people, immunosenescence is characterized by alterations in the composition of lymphocyte populations, blunted or dysregulated immune response to pathogens, pathogen-associated molecular patterns or vaccinations, and a generalized proinflammatory state.[1] Immunosenescence is considered an important risk factor for morbidity and mortality of the aged, contributing to development of many afflictions of the elderly, including neoplastic, inflammatory, and degenerative diseases. Furthermore, an increased susceptibility to infectious pathogens and a decreased response to vaccines designed to protect against infection are commonly observed in the aged. Albeit limited, current evidence suggests that horses likely undergo similar age-related changes in immune function as that observed in people.

Studies of age-associated changes to immune function are plagued by a unique set of confounders, and as a result, data among the studies are often contradictory.

Department of Physiological Sciences, Center of Veterinary Health Sciences, 264 McElroy Hall, Stillwater, OK 74078, USA
E-mail address: diannem@okstate.edu

Vet Clin Equine 32 (2016) 333–341
http://dx.doi.org/10.1016/j.cveq.2016.04.009
0749-0739/16/$ – see front matter
vetequine.theclinics.com

For example, the definition of what age constitutes "aged" is arbitrary, yet critical in study design. If horses are enrolled too young, age-associated changes may not yet have occurred. If enrollment is limited to the extremely old, there may be a selection bias for those animals that have survived to extreme old age in part due to exceptional immune function.[2] If the goal of the study is to identify how immune function becomes defective and leads to increased risk of disease in the aged, those with exceptional aging may not be appropriate. In geriatric horses, often actual age is not known, but estimated from dental wear, a process known to be highly inaccurate.[3] In the elderly, the presence of undiagnosed or subclinical disease is common and may have an impact on immune response.[4] Endocrine and metabolic abnormalities frequently affect old horses, and can be strong influencers of immune function.[5]

AGE-ASSOCIATED CHANGES IN IMMUNE FUNCTION
Cell Populations

Age-associated alterations in lymphocyte subset populations have been documented in several species including people, dogs, and rodents.[6–9] The most consistent change associated with age is a decrease in the number of naïve T cells (CD45RA), which has been documented in aged people, nonhuman primates, and rodents.[10–13] The decrease in naïve T cells has been postulated to be the result of thymic involution.[14] In addition, it has been suggested the loss of naïve T cells may be a consequence of chronic antigenic stimulation.[15,16] Immune response to lifelong latent infections by viruses, especially cytomegalovirus (CMV), are believed to contribute to depletion of the naïve lymphocyte pool.[17,18] Concurrent with the loss of naïve T cells, clonal expansion of CD8 memory cells specific for cytomegalovirus have been observed in the elderly.[18] Furthermore, CMV infection of specific pathogen-free mice was shown to reduce antiviral T-cell responses, reduce vaccination efficiency, and accelerate accumulation of effector memory CD8 T cells, lending direct evidence that exposure to pathogens can restructure the immune system, even in the absence of disease.[19] Due to a lack of available antibodies that can differentiate equine naïve from memory cells, changes in naïve T-cell populations have not been directly examined in the aging horse.

Other findings in human leukocyte populations include alterations in the total number of lymphocytes, CD4, CD8, and B cells. CD4/CD8 ratio, an indicator of an inflammatory versus immunosuppressive bias, has been reported to be altered in human geriatric populations.[20–22] Several studies have investigated lymphocyte populations in aged horses and ponies.[23–27] The total number of lymphocytes, CD4, CD8, and B cells all decrease in aged horses.[23–27] Total lymphocyte percentage also decreases, whereas the percentage of CD4 lymphocytes increases.[25,26] CD4/CD8 ratio was found to be increased in aged horses,[25] suggesting a proinflammatory state occurs in old horses as in aged people.

Cytokine and Acute-Phase Protein Profiles in the Aged Horse

Serum cytokine profiles in aged people typically favor a proinflammatory phenotype.[28,29] Aged horses also show similar cytokine profiles with increased gene expression of tumor necrosis factor (TNF)-α, interleukin (IL)-6, IL-1β, IL-8, interferon (IFN)-γ, IL-15, and IL-18,[26,30] and increased proinflammatory/anti-inflammatory cytokine ratios, including IL-6/IL-10 and TNF-α/IL-10.[30] When cytokine concentration was examined at the protein rather than gene expression level, serum cytokine concentration of TNF-α was increased in aged horses in one study[26] but not another.[30] Several confounding factors might affect serum TNF-α concentration, including concurrent illness, obesity, inflammation, or season of sample collection. The role of other serum cytokines in geriatric horses has not been extensively examined. Although once limited by the lack of availability of reagents validated for use with equine samples, several newer cytokine and acute-phase protein assays are now available and further work needs to be performed to better understand the role of inflammation in healthy aging in horses. Without such data, the potential for age to confound studies of inflammatory biomarkers in various disease states must always be considered.

Immune Responsiveness

Several studies have evaluated the impact of aging on the responsiveness of equine peripheral blood mononuclear cells (PBMCs) following ex vivo immune stimulation.[26,27,30] In people and primates, inflammatory response after stimulation of whole blood or PBMCs from the aged results in a greater release of proinflammatory cytokines than that observed in adults.[31,32] Similarly, ex vivo stimulation of equine PBMCs reveals an increase in TNF-α and IFN-γ production with an increase in age.[26,27,30]

Lymphocyte Function

A consistent finding from studies in both aged rodents and people is a decrease in lymphocyte proliferation. Although a decrease in serum IL-2 concentration or IL-2 receptor expression has been associated with the poor proliferative response observed in the aged,[12,33,34] impairment also has been reported independent of these 2 factors, suggesting intracellular signaling defects also may occur with age.[35] Horses also experience an age-associated decrease in lymphocyte proliferation.[24,26,36] In at least one study, the decrease in proliferation was nonresponsive to IL-2 supplementation and not associated with a change in lymphocyte IL-2 receptor expression.[24] This suggests that in the horse, the age-associated defect in lymphocyte division may be a consequence of alterations in intracellular signaling.

Neutrophil Function

Although immunosenescence affects primarily adaptive immunity, specifically T-cell function, changes in innate immunity occur as well. Innate immunity includes the response of neutrophils and macrophages as a first-line defense against pathogens. Age-associated changes in neutrophil function reported in people and rodents include decreases in phagocytosis, oxidative burst, chemokinesis, and chemotaxis.[37–40] Neutrophil numbers appear to be maintained in the aged,[37–40] although Liu and colleagues[41] reported that in extremely old women a decrease in neutrophil count was associated with functional disability, whereas Fernandez-Garrido and others[42] reported an increase in neutrophil count with frailty. In rodents, age-associated changes in neutrophil function have been associated with increased susceptibility to *Pseudomonas* pneumonia.[43] Although old mice had a greater concentration of pulmonary chemokines, neutrophil count in the airways was markedly lower than that of young mice following infection with *Pseudomonas*, indicating a failure in neutrophil chemotaxis occurred with age. In healthy aged horses, neutrophil adhesion, oxidative burst, and phagocytosis were all found to be unchanged, whereas chemotaxis was increased compared with that of healthy adult horses.[44] The significance of these findings on disease susceptibility in the aged horse is at this time unclear.

In contrast to healthy aged horses, data suggest aged horses with pituitary pars intermedia dysfunction (PPID) have impaired neutrophil function, perhaps contributing to the increased frequency of bacterial diseases, such as abscesses and sinusitis, observed in horses with this disease.[44] Because of the difficulty making an early diagnosis of PPID, it may be necessary to consider all aged horses at higher risk for neutrophil impairment unless proven otherwise.

CLINICAL CONSEQUENCES OF IMMUNOSENESCENCE IN HORSES
Risk of Infectious Disease

Although statements suggesting aged horses are at greater risk for contracting infectious diseases are found throughout the nonscientific literature, very few controlled studies actually document an increased incidence of infectious disease in geriatric horses. Several epidemiologic studies of morbidity and mortality of aged horses have been published recently using a variety of approaches to gather data, including owner surveys, veterinary examinations, retrospective analysis of medical records of referral hospitals, and retrospective analysis of pathology reports.[45–49] Infectious disease was an uncommon cause of disease and death in all of these studies. Despite the suggestion that such conditions as strangles, endoparasitism, or influenza are more common in geriatric horses, to the author's knowledge these assertions remain unsubstantiated.

Although an age-related increase in risk of infection may be the exception rather than the rule, there are examples of diseases that appear to occur more commonly or may be more severe in aged horses. West Nile virus infection may cause more severe disease in geriatric horses compared with adults, as studies have reported a higher case-fatality rate in aged horses.[50,51] Similarly, when horses were experimentally infected with a neuropathogenic strain of equine herpesvirus-1, aged horses appear more susceptible to develop neurologic signs.[52]

In contrast, endoparasite shedding does not appear to be affected by age, although this observation is based on a single, relatively small study with several limitations.[53] Ideally, endoparasite load should be assessed by performing worm counts at postmortem, a highly laborious method that necessitates the study be terminal, not by fecal egg count alone, as performed in this study. Furthermore, fecal egg counts would best be evaluated during peak parasite shedding season. Despite the limitations of the study, greater fecal egg counts were observed in aged horses with PPID compared with that of young horses or healthy aged horses. Therefore, it is important to do quantitative fecal egg counts when performing routine health care of aged horses, as early PPID is often an elusive diagnosis.

Vaccine Responsiveness

A major concern regarding immune decline in the geriatric population is the failure of the aged to develop adequate titers following vaccination, most notably after influenza virus immunization.[54] The inability to elicit protective immunoglobulin levels leads to high morbidity and mortality due to influenza infection in the very old. The response of aged horses to influenza vaccines has also been reported to be less robust than that of young or adult horses in several studies.[36,55,56] Horohov and colleagues[36] reported a 10-fold decrease in resultant titers in aged ponies, compared with adults. Using a different vaccine, Muirhead and colleagues[55] reported a decrease in immunoglobulin (Ig) subtypes IgGa and IgGb in aged horses, although vaccination of both adults and aged horses resulted in what is considered to be a protective titer. However, challenge studies to evaluate clinical outcomes in aged horses following conventional vaccination for influenza or other diseases have not been reported. Thus, the effectiveness of target titers at protecting aged horses from disease is unknown. Regardless of the effectiveness of influenza vaccine in aged horses, an increased incidence of influenza infection in geriatric horses has not been reported.

Response to naïve antigenic challenge was also examined in horses older than 20 years. Contrary to what has been reported in primates,[57–59] the magnitude of a primary antibody response did not decline with age.[55] When a rabies vaccine was administered to rabies vaccine–naïve aged horses, the antibody titer after both the initial and second immunization did not differ from that of the nonaged, adult horses. However, in this study, 80% of both the control and aged population had low serum selenium concentrations, which could result in a suboptimal vaccine response in both groups. Further studies are needed to clarify the ability of aged horse to respond to naïve and amnestic vaccine challenge and to assist in the development of ideal vaccination protocol for geriatric horses.

Chronic Inflammatory Diseases

As stated previously, immunosenescence includes age-associated remodeling of the immune system resulting in poor immunity and an exaggerated inflammatory state. Although aged horses appear to generally maintain an adequate protective immunity against pathogens, inflammatory diseases are extremely common in the geriatric equid. It is unclear what role age-associated imbalance in cytokine and acute-phase response (favoring a proinflammatory response) contributes to initiation or progression of the chronic inflammatory diseases that occur in geriatric horses. A better understanding of the interactions between immune changes due solely to age and increased risk of inflammatory disease in the old horse, might lead to development of effective preventive strategies to minimize age-related systemic inflammation and thus delay the onset or minimize the severity of chronic inflammatory diseases in old horses.

SPECIAL CONSIDERATIONS FOR STUDIES IN IMMUNOLOGY OF AGING

Determining the cause of age-induced decline in immune function is complicated. First, it is important to differentiate functional changes that are due to age alone from disease-induced pathology. In an aged population, this can be difficult because of the high prevalence of comorbidities that contribute to chronic, low-grade inflammation. For example, the role of chronic inflammatory diseases (such as osteoarthritis or reactive airway disease) and the effect of chronic or latent pathogens (such as endoparasites or herpes viruses) on systemic immune aging in horses has been largely ignored thus far. Ideally, a strict recruitment protocol should be used when designing studies of the effects of age on immune function. In human immunologic research, a screening procedure known as the SENIEUR protocol has been developed,[2] which combines a history, clinical examination, diagnostic blood work, and urine analyses to identify healthy aged individuals for study inclusion. Adoption of similar standardized protocols in veterinary gerontology may improve the quality of data gathered. In studies of aged horses, it is important to consider gender and hormonal status during the study period, as several of the pituitary and adrenal hormones are strong modifiers of immune function. The profound effect of season on the output of pars intermedia hormones and the high prevalence of PPID in the aged equine population[5,60,61] can markedly confound a study designed to investigate age-specific immune function in horses. Other important considerations when assessing immune function in aged horses include diet, medications and supplements, exercise, travel, and environmental conditions of the study participants.

SUMMARY

There is great interest by the horse-owning community in maintaining horses in optimal health and function into late life. Much remains to be learned regarding interventions designed to preserve a youthful immune system in the old horse popu-lation. Initial data suggest that, unlike people, geriatric horses, in the absence of comorbidities, are relatively effective at avoiding infectious diseases. However, the high prevalence of immunosuppressive endocrine disease (eg, PPID) in aged horses, combined with the difficulty in establishing a diagnosis of early PPID, means that all aged horses should be considered at high risk of poor immune function and treated accordingly. Interventions designed to deter the shift toward a proinflammatory bias that occurs in old horses may provide protection against numerous chronic diseases that limit the health span of horses.

REFERENCES

1. Gruver AL, Hudson LL, Sempowski GD. Immunosenescence of ageing. J Pathol 2007;211:144.
2. Sansoni P, Vescovini R, Fagnoni F, et al. The immune system in extreme longevity. Exp Gerontol 2008;43:61.
3. Muylle S, Simoens P, Lauwers H. Ageing horses by an examination of their incisor teeth: an (im)possible task? Vet Rec 1996;138:295–301.
4. Ligthart GJ, Corberand JX, Fournier C, et al. Admission criteria for immunogeron-tological studies in man: the SENIEUR protocol. Mech Ageing Dev 1984;28:47.
5. McGowan TW, Pinchbeck GP, McGowan CM. Prevalence, risk factors and clinical signs predictive for equine pituitary pars intermedia dysfunction in aged horses. Equine Vet J 2012;45:74–9.
6. Sansoni P, Cossarizza A, Brianti V, et al. Lymphocyte subsets and natural killer cell activity in healthy old people and centenarians. Blood 1993;82:2767.
7. Greeley EH, Kealy RD, Ballam JM, et al. The influence of age on the canine immune system. Vet Immunol Immunopathol 1996;55:1.
8. Watabe A, Fukumoto S, Komatsu T, et al. Alterations of lymphocyte subpopula-tions in healthy dogs with aging and in dogs with cancer. Vet Immunol Immuno-pathol 2011;142:189.
9. Maue AC, Yager EJ, Swain SL, et al. T-cell immunosenescence: lessons learned from mouse models of aging. Trends Immunol 2009;30:301.
10. Lazuardi L, Jenewein B, Wolf AM, et al. Age-related loss of naïve T cells and dys-regulation of T-cell/B-cell interactions in human lymph nodes. Immunology 2005; 114:37–43.
11. Naylor K, Li G, Vallejo AN, et al. The influence of age on T cell generation and TCR diversity. J Immunol 2005;174:7446.
12. Rea IM, Stewart M, Campbell P, et al. Changes in lymphocyte subsets, interleukin 2, and soluble interleukin 2 receptor in old and very old age. Gerontology 1996; 42:69.
13. Ferrando-Martinez S, Ruiz-Mateos E, Hernandez A, et al. Age-related deregula-tion of naive T cell homeostasis in elderly humans. Age (Dordr) 2011;33:197.
14. Pawelec G, Adibzadeh M, Solana R, et al. The T cell in the ageing individual. Mech Ageing Dev 1997;93:35–45.
15. Lang A, Nikolich-Zugich J. Functional CD8 T cell memory responding to persis-tent latent infection is maintained for life. J Immunol 2011;187:3759.
16. Fulop T, Larbi A, Pawelec G. Human T cell aging and the impact of persistent viral infections. Front Immunol 2013;4:271.
17. Pawelec G, Derhovanessian E. Role of CMV in immune senescence. Virus Res 2011;157:175.

18. Ouyang Q, Wagner WM, Wikby A, et al. Large numbers of dysfunctional CD8+ T lymphocytes bearing receptors for a single dominant CMV epitope in the very old. J Clin Immunol 2003;23:247–57.

19. Mekker A, Tchang VS, Haeberli L, et al. Immune senescence: relative contributions of age and cytomegalovirus infection. PLoS Pathog 2012;8:e1002850.

20. Hodkinson CF, O'Connor JM, Alexander HD, et al. Whole blood analysis of phagocytosis, apoptosis, cytokine production, and leukocyte subsets in healthy older men and women: the ZENITH study. J Gerontol A Biol Sci Med Sci 2006; 61:907.

21. Peres A, Bauer M, da Cruz IB, et al. Immunophenotyping and T-cell proliferative capacity in a healthy aged population. Biogerontology 2003;4:289.

22. Huppert FA, Pinto EM, Morgan K, et al. Survival in a population sample is predicted by proportions of lymphocyte subsets. Mech Ageing Dev 2003;124:449.

23. Ralston SL, Nockels CF, Squires EL. Differences in diagnostic test results and hematologic data between aged and young horses. Am J Vet Res 1988;49:1387.

24. Horohov DW, Kydd JH, Hannant D. The effect of aging on T cell responses in the horse. Dev Comp Immunol 2002;26:121.

25. McFarlane D, Sellon DC, Gibbs SA. Age-related quantitative alterations in lymphocyte subsets and immunoglobulin isotypes in healthy horses. Am J Vet Res 2001;62:1413.

26. Adams AA, Breathnach CC, Katepalli MP, et al. Advanced age in horses affects divisional history of T cells and inflammatory cytokine production. Mech Ageing Dev 2008;129:656.

27. Schnabel CL, Steinig P, Schberth HJ, et al. Influences of age and sex on leukocytes of healthy horses and their ex vivo cytokine release. Vet Immunol Immunopathol 2015;165:64–74.

28. Forsey RJ, Thompson JM, Ernerudh J, et al. Plasma cytokine profiles in elderly humans. Mech Ageing Dev 2003;124:487.

29. Leng SX, Yang H, Walston JD. Decreased cell proliferation and altered cytokine production in frail older adults. Aging Clin Exp Res 2004;16:249.

30. McFarlane D, Holbrook TC. Cytokine dysregulation in aged horses and horses with pituitary pars intermedia dysfunction. J Vet Intern Med 2008;22:436.

31. Eylar EH, Molina F, Quinones C, et al. Comparison of mitogenic responses of young and old rhesus monkey T cells to lectins and interleukins 2 and 4. Cell Immunol 1989;121:328.

32. Gabriel P, Cakman I, Rink L. Overproduction of monokines by leukocytes after stimulation with lipopolysaccharide in the elderly. Exp Gerontol 2002;37:235.

33. Chopra RK, Powers DC, Kendig NE, et al. Soluble interleukin 2 receptors released from mitogen stimulated human peripheral blood lymphocytes bind interleukin 2 and inhibit IL2 dependent cell proliferation. Immunol Invest 1989;18:961.

34. Weigle WO. Effects of aging on the immune system. Hosp Pract (Off Ed) 1989;24: 112–9.

35. Song L, Kim YH, Chopra RK, et al. Age-related effects in T cell activation and proliferation. Exp Gerontol 1993;28:313.

36. Horohov DW, Dimock A, Guirnalda P, et al. Effect of exercise on the immune response of young and old horses. Am J Vet Res 1999;60:643.

37. Schroder AK, Rink L. Neutrophil immunity of the elderly. Mech Ageing Dev 2003; 124:419.

38. Peters T, Weiss JM, Sindrilaru A, et al. Reactive oxygen intermediate-induced pathomechanisms contribute to immunosenescence, chronic inflammation and autoimmunity. Mech Ageing Dev 2009;130:564.

39. Lord JM, Butcher S, Killampali V, et al. Neutrophil ageing and immunesenescence. Mech Ageing Dev 2001;122:1521.
40. Solana R, Tarazona R, Gayoso I, et al. Innate immunosenescence: effect of aging on cells and receptors of the innate immune system in humans. Semin Immunol 2012;24:331.
41. Liu Z, Wang Y, Huang J, et al. Blood biomarkers and functional disability among extremely longevous individuals: a population-based study. J Gerontol A Biol Sci Med Sci 2015;70:623–7.
42. Fernandez-Garrido J, Navarro-Martinez R, Buiques-Gonzalez C, et al. The value of neutrophil and lymphocyte count in frail older women. Exp Gerontol 2014;54: 35–41.
43. Chen MM, Palmer JL, Plackett TP, et al. Age-related differences in the neutrophil response to pulmonary pseudomonas infection. Exp Gerontol 2014;54:42–6.
44. McFarlane D, Hill K, Anton J. Neutrophil function in healthy aged horses and horses with pituitary dysfunction. Vet Immunol Immunopathol 2015;165:99–106.
45. Silva AG, Furr MO. Diagnoses, clinical pathology findings and treatment outcome of geriatric horses: 345 cases (2006-2010). J Am Vet Med Assoc 2013;243:17.
46. Ireland JL, Clegg PD, McGowan CM, et al. Factors associated with mortality of geriatric horses in the United Kingdom. Prev Vet Med 2011;101:204–18.
47. Williams N. Disease conditions in geriatric horses. Equine Disease Quarterly 2000;8. Available at: http://www2.ca.uky.edu/gluck/q/2000/jan00/Q_jan00.htm.
48. Brosnahan MM, Paradis MR. Demographics and clinical characteristics of geriatric horses. 467 cases (1989-1999). J Am Vet Med Assoc 2003;223:93–8.
49. McGowan TW, Pinchbeck G, Phillips CJ, et al. A survey of aged horses in Queensland, Australia. Part 2: clinical signs and owners perceptions of health and welfare. Aust Vet J 2010;88:465–71.
50. Schuler LA, Khaitsa ML, Dyer NW, et al. Evaluation of an outbreak of West Nile virus infection in horses: 569 cases (2001). J Am Vet Med Assoc 2004;225: 1084–9.
51. Salazer P, Traub-Dargatz JL, Morley PS, et al. Outcome of equids with clinical signs of West Mile virus infection and factors associated with death. J Am Vet Med Assoc 2004;225:267–74.
52. Allen GP. Risk factors for development of neurologic disease after experimental exposure to equine herpesvirus-1 in horses. Am J Vet Res 2008;69:1595–600.
53. McFarlane D, Hale GM, Johnson EM, et al. Fecal egg counts after anthelmintic administration to aged horses and horses with pituitary pars intermedia dysfunction. J Am Vet Med Assoc 2010;236:330–4.
54. Reber AJ, Chirkova T, Kim JH, et al. Immunosenescence and challenges of vaccination against influenza in the aging population. Aging Dis 2012;3:68.
55. Muirhead TL, McClure JT, Wichtel JJ, et al. The effect of age on serum antibody titers after rabies and influenza vaccination in healthy horses. J Vet Intern Med 2008;22:654.
56. Adams AA, Sturgill TL, Breathnach CC, et al. Humoral and cell-mediated immune responses of old horses following recombinant canarypox virus vaccination and subsequent challenge infections. Vet Immunol Immunopathol 2011;139:128–40.
57. Cicin-Sain L, Smyk-Pearson S, Currier N, et al. Loss of naive T cells and repertoire constriction predict poor response to vaccination in old primates. J Immunol 2010;184:6739.
58. Smith TP, Kennedy SL, Fleshner M. Influence of age and physical activity on the primary in vivo antibody and T cell-mediated responses in men. J Appl Physiol 2004;97:491.

59. Aberle JH, Stiasny K, Kundi M, et al. Mechanistic insights into the impairment of memory B cells and antibody production in the elderly. Age 2013;35:371–81.
60. McFarlane D, Donaldson MT, McDonnell SM, et al. Effects of season and sample handling on measurement of plasma alpha-melanocyte-stimulating hormone concentrations in horses and ponies. Am J Vet Res 2004;65:1463–8.
61. Donaldson MT, McDonnell SM, Schanbacher BJ, et al. Variation in plasma adrenocorticotropic hormone concentration and dexamethasone suppression test results with season, age, and sex in healthy ponies and horses. J Vet Intern Med 2005;19:217–22.

Nutritional Management of the Older Horse

Caroline McG. Argo, BSc, BVSc, PhD, MRCVS

KEYWORDS

- Horse • Aged • Geriatric • Nutrition • PPID • Obesity • Weight loss

KEY POINTS

- Health in old age is promoted by good health throughout life.
- Older horses that remain in good health but are losing body condition may benefit from "senior" diets—but rule out other causes of weight loss first.
- Obesity is common in older horses.
- The imposition of corrective management is important.
- Nutritional provision for older, failing animals should be regularly reappraised to compensate for advancing feeding and digestive dysfunction.

INTRODUCTION

Recent years have evidenced a shift in the demographics of horse and pony ownership, away from primary working roles and toward companion animal status. In the United Kingdom, leisure animals now account for approximately 60% of the national equine herd, and similar trends are reported for other industrialized nations.[1] This leisure classification encompasses a broad spectrum of animals, ranging from pets and companions, to those participating at relatively high levels of nonprofessional competitive events. Leisure animals now dominate the equine sector, whereas relatively few are maintained primarily for the economic benefit of the owner, but all clearly occupy important societal roles. It is likely that this shift in equine ownership is permanent and set to increase, both numerically and geographically.

Accessibility to horse ownership has greatly expanded to include a welcome involvement of many people new to animal management. This change in ownership has been accompanied by a decrease in individual animal workloads, improved veterinary support, and increased emotional and economic investments in individual animal care. Not surprisingly, these changes have promoted longevity among horses and

Disclosure Statement: The author recognizes no sources of conflicting interest.
Department of Veterinary Clinical Sciences, School of Veterinary Medicine, Faculty of Health and Medical Sciences, University of Surrey, Main Building, Manor Park Campus, Daphne Jackson Road, Guildford GU2 7AL, UK
E-mail address: c.argo@surrey.ac.uk

Vet Clin Equine 32 (2016) 343–354
http://dx.doi.org/10.1016/j.cveq.2016.04.010   vetequine.theclinics.com
0749-0739/16/$ – see front matter © 2016 Elsevier Inc. All rights reserved.

ponies, with older animals being maintained beyond their functionally useful lifespans.[2,3]

However, not all of the welfare implications associated with these changes have been beneficial. A lessening of economic constraints and performance expectations has served to uncouple animal management from traditional wisdoms in agriculture and nutrition. The number and variety of concentrate feedstuffs targeted specifically at the aged horse, combined with uncertainty about exactly when age-related dietary changes should be introduced, have created a great deal of confusion among horse owners, managers, and veterinarians alike.[4] Education in the management of this emotionally important, aged animal cohort has failed to keep pace with the needs of this new ownership demographic.

AGE-RELATED CHANGES THAT IMPACT ON FEEDING AND DIGESTIVE FUNCTION

"Old age rarely comes alone." The spectrum and rate of onset of age-related impairments in function are largely dictated by the cumulative effects of genetic and epigenetic endowments, environmental, health, work, and lifestyle–related factors acquired across the lifetime of the animal.[5] Aging in otherwise healthy horses, as in other mammals, will inexorably lead to the eventual presentation of senescent changes. These changes include sarcopenia, the loss of body mass (BM), and the onset of organ dysfunction with progressive attrition of the dental, neural, immunologic, and other systems.[5] For the horse, the age-related onset of progressive pituitary pars intermedia dysfunction (PPID) might be considered an individually variable accelerant of the aging process, which further compromises body function.[6]

Body Composition and Aging

Skeletal muscle can account for 40% of BM and 60% of maintenance energy requirements in healthy animals.[7] In man, changes in body composition with aging favor fat accumulation in adipose tissues and muscle at the expense of lean muscle mass.[5] Lehnhard and coworkers[8] compared the body composition of aged (>20 years) and young (4–8 years) Standardbred mares to suggest similar trends in horses. Data in this study used the formula presented by Kane and colleagues[9] to estimate body fat and, by extrapolation, fat-free mass, based on measures of rump fat depth. Although the accuracy of this method has since been questioned, empirical observations of geriatric horses and ponies would support this finding.[10]

The regional distribution of superficially palpable adipose tissues throughout the body is significantly altered with advanced age and more markedly with overlying PPID.[11] However, a questionnaire study (73% response rate) of owners who owned at least one horse over the age of 20 years indicated that most old (68%, 111/165) and young (64%, 34/52) horses were considered to be in moderate or good body condition score (BCS = 2–3/5) by their owners.[12] Although there is a general expectation that older horses tend to thinness, only 4% (7/165) of these older animals were reported as being in poor or very poor (BCS = 0–1/5) body condition. Conversely, 28% (47/165) of the aged horses were considered fat or very fat (BCS = 4–5/5), a prevalence of obesity statistically indistinguishable from the younger animal cohort (34%, 18/52).[12] That horses 15 years of age or older were just as likely to be reported by their owners as overweight/obese (10.5%) as underweight (8%) was confirmed in a study of UK pleasure horses.[13]

Thermoregulation may become less efficient in older horses, as a consequence of reduced BM, adipose tissue redistribution, and alterations in fluid compartmentalization.[14] Less efficient thermoregulation suggests that precautions are needed to avoid excessive heat loss or gain across the body surface in winter and summer, respectively.[15] Impairment of immunologic function may also render aged horses at risk of subclinical disease and increased endoparasitism. As hepatic function decreases with advanced old age, catabolic processes start to outstrip anabolic activities, and the normal dynamic turnover of tissues (most visibly muscle and bone) starts to fail. These changes, combined with decreased activity in older animals, might be predicted to reduce metabolic energy requirements in older animals.[16]

Food Intake

There can be an acceptance by owners that weight loss in their older animals is an inevitable consequence of age-related senescence, and this can disincline owners from seeking interventions or veterinary advice. Recent epidemiologic research that followed up owner questionnaires with veterinary evaluation of individual aged horses ($\geq$15 years and $\geq$30 years) identified a clear underrecognition of concurrent disease.[17,18]

Food intake tends to diminish as animals age.[5] Age-related decreased food intake can be multifactorial. Care is needed to determine possible causes in individual animals and their circumstances. Decreased appetite in older animals can be associated with a primary reduction in the ability or willingness to eat or can be secondary to decreased metabolic demands. Energy requirements can decrease as older animals become less active and lose BM, and the maintenance demands of altered muscle metabolism decline as a consequence of sarcopenic and muscle fiber type changes.[8]

Anorexia with consequent weight loss can often be directly related to dental or musculoskeletal disease, or where animals are maintained in group situations, a reduction of social hierarchy. Decreased fiber digestibility has been noted in older animals, and long fibers and whole cereal may be seen in the feces.[19] Given the hypsodont nature of their dentition, dental insufficiency is ultimately an unavoidable component of aging in horses.[20] Senile diastema, periodontal disease, loss of effective occlusal surfaces, and frank tooth loss all serve to reduce effective food intake and mastication to a point at which maintenance requirements are not met.[20,21]

Regrettably, community care for the elderly is unknown to the equine population! Studies of feral horse and pony breeds maintained under domestic or range conditions indicate that older animals can lose their position in the social hierarchy at pasture and are frequently bullied and prevented from grazing or accessing group feeding stations, especially where the availability of feedstuffs is limited.[22–27] A recent study of 194 outdoor-living domestic horses maintained as 42 separate herds provided further evidence to indicate that, while dominance demonstrated a quadratic relationship with age, the relationship between BCS and age was much stronger.[28] Conversely, dominant animals were at higher risk of obesity.[28] These studies reinforce the importance of maintaining body condition in elderly animals and highlight the vulnerability that animals may experience with increasing frailty. Musculoskeletal disease is common in the older horse. Of 467 aged (>20 years) horses referred to a veterinary hospital, 24% were presented for the evaluation of musculoskeletal disease. Of the 80 for which evaluations were available, 44% had foot lesions, 86% of which were laminitis, and 40% had osteoarthritis or degenerative joint disease.[29] The investigators reported that very old horses were less likely to be presented for lameness evaluation, and that this may reflect decreased work demands. However, orthopedic pain can add considerably to an animal's unwillingness to eat, especially at pasture or where it must compete with peers for forage.

The Gastrointestinal Microbiome and Nutrient Digestibility

The combination of increased stress, reduced time spent feeding, difficulties in prehension and mastication, and decreased salivary production associated with decreased chewing are additive. Older animals are more prone to choke and impaction colic, and the increased length of swallowed fiber decreases nutrient digestibility, which may initiate undesirable changes to the hind gut microflora. An altered microflora is unlikely to synthesize B complex and K vitamins effectively, and although usually subclinical, signs of specific deficiencies may be present.[4]

The digestion of plant fiber to yield short-chain fatty acids, important metabolic substrates for horses, depends on the microflora within the hindgut.[30] Age has a marked impact on the bacterial diversity within the human gastrointestinal tract[31] with clear alterations in the abundance of some species (decreased: *Bacteroidetes*, *Clostridia*, and *Bifidibacteria*; increased: *Proteobacteria* and *Bacilli*).[31–33] In horses, the fecal microbiota has been shown to be representative of the microflora inhabiting the major fiber-fermenting regions of the distal hindgut (right dorsal colon to rectum).[34,35]

In man, aging is associated with a narrowing of bacterial diversity in the gastrointestinal tract, which may be associated with primary changes in digestive and metabolic functions.[31,36] When the fecal microbiome of mature (n = 8, 5–12 years) and elderly stock-horse mares (n = 9, 19–28 years) were compared, Dougal and coworkers[30] recorded a comparable reduction in the bacterial diversity of equine feces with increased age. Given the importance of the hindgut microbiome on the digestion of dietary fiber, it was noteworthy that age-related alterations in bacterial diversity were not accompanied by measurable differences in the apparent digestibility of any macronutrient or mineral evaluated.[37]

Despite this evidence that digestive efficiency appears unaltered by age in healthy horses, many compounded senior horse diets contain extruded or finely ground cereals to improve fiber digestibility, increased concentrations of crude protein (12%–16%), phosphorous (0.45%–0.5%), and reduced calcium (<1%). Evidence for these products dates from a 1980s study that compared geriatric horses (>20 years) with younger animals. Older animals had reduced phosphorous absorption and protein and fiber digestibilities. Plasma concentrations of vitamin C (ascorbic acid) were also reduced in the older animals.[19] However, studies performed over a decade later by the same and other research groups failed to demonstrate any clear requirement to alter nutritional provision for otherwise healthy Standardbred geriatric horses.[37,38] The investigators of the original study hypothesized that the nutritional impairment measured in the 1980s was most probably related to chronic scarring of the gut mucosa as a result of life-long endoparasitism and uncorrected, abnormal dentition. Similarly managed, elderly horses (20–33 years) had higher fecal strongyle egg counts than mature animals (5–15 years).[39] The importance of appropriately managed endoparasitism in older horses as a key component in the preservation of their digestive efficiency is noteworthy. However, older animals are susceptible to reinfection, and rigorous anthelmintic regimens should be pursued.

It should be emphasized that although the digestive efficiency of mature, healthy animals would appear to be unaltered by age alone, the impact of chronic disease and ultimate senescent changes on nutrient digestibility are likely to be both marked and diverse.

Pituitary Pars Intermedia Dysfunction

Increasing age is a significant risk factor for the development of PPID.[40] Although the onset of PPID is often unnoticed and difficult to determine,[11] studies of referral hospital and primary care cases indicated that the typical age of owner recognition of clinically apparent PPID was between 19 and 21 years of age for referral cases[41–47] compared with field-based epidemiologic studies, where a younger age of detection of 15 years and older was found.[40] The difference between the age of presentation is largely due to owner underrecognition of clinical signs of PPID, which in the past have been attributed to age-related senescence.

Overproduction of proopiomelanocortin peptides in PPID cases are considered to be the primary cause of metabolic disturbances associated with the condition.[11] Progressive changes in the relative proportions of fat and muscle are a major presenting sign of this condition.[11] Sarcopenia can be marked, whereas relative body fat content may increase. Superficially visible adipose tissues may be subject to redistribution away from the abdominothoracic regions and toward the nuchal crest and dorsal rump/loin. Altered fat patterning with an unquantified element of lypodystrophy is also evident with hypercorticism in man and other mammals.[48] Skeletal muscle and adipose tissues are the most labile of the body's energy reserves. Alterations in their relative distribution may have marked implications for energy metabolism and nutrition, but the extent to which these changes are also accompanied by perturbations in energy and protein metabolism is relatively unknown. These considerations have marked implications for the nutritional management of the PPID case. Until the functionality of altered adipose tissues is more fully understood, the application of standard BCS systems to assess nutrient status should be applied with caution for older horses. BCS systems were primarily developed to appraise total flesh cover in food animals before later being validated for the evaluation of adiposity in healthy horses.[49,50] Further work is needed to develop meaningful BCS systems for PPID and geriatric animals and to understand the functional relationships between PPID-associated body composition changes and whole animal energetics.

DEFINING THE ELDERLY HORSE

Health in old age is promoted by appropriate nutrition, exercise, and welfare in early life. In contrast to the working animals of yesteryear, today's horses and ponies generally enter old-age having enjoyed a relatively disease-free, low-stress life, with a gut untroubled by scarring associated with chronic parasitism. However, the multiplicity of owners throughout a horse's lifetime can mean that the guardians of old age often lack useful histories. The chronology of aging differs remarkably between individuals, and this reinforces the need to evaluate each animal independently.[2] Data from the United States suggest that horses are perceived to be elderly at around 22 years of age, while 40% of owners of horses aged 15 years and over had already made age-related changes to their animal's nutrient provision.[12]

For nutritional purposes, older horses (>20 years) can generally be categorized aged-normal (healthy animals that may be normally overweight or underweight), or geriatric, a term reserved for older horses with clear signs of senescent changes alone or in the company of concurrent disease, which may include PPID.

MONITORING THE ELDERLY HORSE

Until the point at which the health of older individuals begins to be compromised by the onset of senescent changes, there may be no indication to make specific alterations to nutritional provision—other than those linked to their ever-decreasing workload and the need to maintain an ideal body weight. However, there is a clear case that horses in their 20s and beyond benefit from frequent monitoring to identify, address, and ameliorate the inevitable onset of age-related "disease."

Veterinarians should work with owners to develop protocols for animal care and monitoring. Care regimens should include robust anthelmintic treatments, foot and dental care, and appropriate management of any musculoskeletal pain. Where animals are kept at pasture, owners should be alert for signs of bullying and be prepared to alter pasture groupings to minimize stress and feeding completion or control pasture intakes. A decrease in the animal's capacity to thermoregulate warrants constant and ever-changing support in the form of appropriate rugging, stabling, and clipping. Nutritional advice should promote the maintenance of ideal body condition (see later discussion). All animals should receive appropriate daily quantities of a vitamin and mineral product designed to complement their diets.

Given the likelihood and severity of laminitis in the elderly horse population, it is justifiable that all animals older than 20 years of age should be screened annually or biannually to monitor insulin sensitivity and serum adrenocorticotropin concentrations as a predictive marker of PPID. Owners should be directed on how to monitor BCS, and animals should be weighed and/or the belly girth circumference (widest point of the abdomen) measured fortnightly as a proxy for weight change. Consistent recordings should objectively highlight change and the need for intervention.

NUTRITIONAL MANAGEMENT OF OLDER HORSES
The Normal Elderly Horse that Is Losing Condition

Weight loss in older horses can be multifactorial and should be investigated with an open mind. Common causes of weight loss in older animals can often be attributed to pain, bullying at pasture (a self-fulfilling prophecy as social dominance is positively associated with BCS and negatively with age[28]), chronic parasitism, poor dental health, or inadequate nutritional provision. Identification and correction of these factors should allow a progressive return to normal condition with minimal adjustment to standard nutritional regimes. Failure to respond to corrective therapy may indicate the onset of senescent changes or disease, and veterinary and nutritional advice for the geriatric horse might be beneficial.

The Normal Obese Elderly Horse

Older horses will have decreasing basal metabolic rates. Appetite in healthy aged horses can exceed maintenance requirements, promoting positive energy balance and fat deposition. It is important to distinguish the truly obese animal from one demonstrating PPID-associated adipose tissue redistribution. Obesity in older horses should be managed aggressively. Animals in this age group may be at heightened risk of obesity-related morbidities and disease. Old age, obesity, and PPID are all risk factors for insulin resistance, and in combination, these factors increase the likelihood of acute and chronic laminitis.

The restoration of normal body weight in obese animals begins with a full clinical examination to record baseline values against which corrective progress can be appraised. Outset measures include BCS, direct or indirect measures/estimates of BM (kg), belly girth (cm), and a dynamic evaluation of insulin/glucose dynamics. The presence of insulin resistance will influence forage selections for weight loss.[51–53] Environment and nutritional management should be appraised. All supplementary feeding of concentrate feedstuffs should be terminated and substituted for an appropriate daily quantity of a mineral/vitamin supplement tailored to complement a forage diet.

Weight loss at pasture

Controlled weight loss is best accomplished with the animal housed away from pasture. Where removal from pasture is not possible, grazing can be restricted by strip-grazing or with the judicious use of grazing muzzles, which restrict as opposed to prevent intake.[54] The successful use of muzzles can be onerous and problematic. It should be confirmed that the animal has learned to drink while wearing the muzzle. Animals should be inspected, and muzzles should be removed periodically to permit self and social grooming. Grass ingestion is difficult to quantify. Where animals can be paddocked individually, fecal output can be a useful proxy for consumption. The successfully graze-restricted animal could generally be expected to produce around half of the fecal mass produced under the same conditions before restriction. Removal of rugs and partial clipping of the winter coat can be effective aids to increasing energy expenditure in winter. Where possible, exercise should be given as an adjunct to dietary restriction.

Weight loss for the stabled horse
Dietary restriction of stabled horses is more readily accomplished and may be essential for the prompt restoration of insulin sensitivity in insulin-resistant animals.[52] Obese insulin-sensitive animals should initially be restricted to 1.25% of BM as daily dry matter (DM) intake of grass hay (~1.5% of BM as fresh grass hay). Provision of a forage balancer product is essential. Daily hay rations should be divided and offered as 2 to 4 meals, ideally using doubled, small-gauge hay nets to prolong time spent feeding.[51]

Because of the potential for rapid body fat mobilization and the increased risk for hyperlipidemia, horses on restricted diets should be carefully monitored, with weekly weight loss targets of between 0.5% and 1.25% of outset BM considered clinically safe.[51,53,55] For practical purposes, 2 points are noteworthy. First, weight loss rates can be highly variable between individuals (±55%).[51,53] Second, hay quality can significantly alter the predicted plane of energy restriction.[51] Where possible, the specific hay batch should be analyzed for DM, nonstructural carbohydrates (NSC), and energy. Ideally, a moderate or poor quality of hay with an NSC (water-soluble carbohydrates [WSC] + starch) content of less than 10% is recommended[56]; however, in many regions, this can only be achieved by soaking hay, where considerations of DM loss during soaking must be taken into consideration (see later discussion).[51]

Weight loss is most marked (~4% of outset BM) during the first week of dietary restriction and then proceeds in a relatively linear manner before it eventually slows as metabolic rate is adaptively suppressed.[53] Weight loss or changes in belly girth measures should be monitored weekly. BCS is a less useful monitor of weight loss because internal adipose tissues (retroperitoneal and visceral) appear to be mobilized preferentially, and significant losses must be incurred before superficial adipose reserves (evaluated by BCS systems) alter appreciably.[53,55]

Monitoring weight loss allows hay provision to be adjusted to compensate for over-rapid weight losses, either as a result of poor hay qualities or where the individual is highly weight-loss sensitive. Conversely, weight loss–resistant animals, which fail to respond to the initial plane of restriction, may require hay provision to be decreased further to 1% of BM daily as hay DM.[53]

Where animals are known to be insulin resistant, soaking hay for 8 to 16 hours can be used to promote weight loss, but this should only be done with veterinary supervision. Feeding soaked hay at 1.25% of BM as DM before soaking doubled the rate of weight loss compared with that of animals that were fed the same proportional amount of hay fed unsoaked. Soaking incurred significant losses in hay DM (~20%) and severely increased degree of negative energy balance imposed (from 81% to 64% of maintenance energy requirements).[51] Both the unsoaked and soaked hay diets resulted in weight loss and improved insulin sensitivity in all animals, but this improvement was more rapid when hay was fed soaked, largely through the leaching of

WSC.[51,52] The impact of soaking on WSC leaching (10%–60%) is highly variable between hay batches, but the extent of mineral losses (20%–60%) dictates that soaked hay must always be fed in conjunction with an appropriate forage balancer.[51,57] It is recommended that client-specific hays are tested to determine the impact of soaking on WSC concentrations and to predict the DM content of soaked hay at the point of feeding.[51]

Postdiet animals will have reduced metabolic energy requirements.[53] When dietary restrictions are eventually relaxed, weight regain is likely.[58] The correction of obesity is a long-term commitment, and the maintenance of an ideal BCS is a life-long endeavor!

THE GERIATRIC HORSE

As animals age, progressive changes can be insidious, and the loss of body condition may go unnoticed until well advanced. Furthermore, conditions such as PPID may promote gradual changes in the distribution and nature of superficial fat deposits. In these older animals, BCS and BM data generated from the use of standard systems and weigh tapes may be misleading and suggestive of radical weight loss.

Evaluation of the animal's clinical presentation, environment, and current nutrition can be revealing. Musculoskeletal pain can prevent animals from feeding effectively from the floor or competing with fitter peers for limited resources.[4] Appropriate analgesia can be rejuvenating, but moving an animal to a separate paddock, ideally with a well-tempered companion, may also be necessary. Separation also allows older animals to receive concentrate feeds apart from field mates, both to remove competition and to allow quantity consumed, ease, and vigor of feeding to be observed.[4]

Grass remains the forage of choice for older animals. Grazing promotes gentle exercise, and the higher water content of fresh grass relative to hay/haylage facilitates mastication (assuming dental compromise), swallowing, and digestion. Many severely dentally compromised animals still benefit from turn out to pasture and will obtain a significant proportion of daily intake provided pasture lengths exceed 6 cm. Soaked, processed complete feeds are greatly valued in the maintenance of these animals.

Compound feedstuffs should be highly palatable and heavily moistened to aid in the prevention of choke and subsequent digestion.[15] Processed (eg, extruded, ground, pelleted) compound feeds are preferred because the smaller particle sizes are more easily masticated, swallowed, and digested, with a reduced risk for impaction colic.[59] Significant improvements in weight gain, BCS, plasma total protein, physical activity levels, and hair condition can be obtained through the feeding of processed feeds to geriatric horses.[60] Compound feeds containing increased crude protein (12%–14% compared with 8.5% for younger mature animals) of greater biological value (ideal amino acid profile) should be selected.

Energy supplementation focusing on diets high in cereal (starch) or WSCs should be discouraged. Many older animals may have undiagnosed insulin resistance as a result of age alone or in combination with PPID. Simple sugars are highly glycemic; dental compromise decreases mastication effort, and grain may pass directly to the hindgut. Both directly increase laminitis risk. Should increased dietary energy provision be indicated, oil (up to 500 mL of vegetable, corn, or soya oil) can be slowly (2–3 weeks) introduced into the diet to great effect.[61]

Most geriatric diets limit calcium to bare maintenance requirements (<1%), whereas phosphorous provision is slightly increased (0.4%–0.65%). Excessive calcium provision to older horses has been linked to an increased incidence of urinary calculi.[62] The inclusion of probiotics or yeast cultures offers a good source of B-complex vitamins to augment synthesis by a potentially impaired microflora.[30]

Nutritional provision for the older animal must be constantly reviewed. Age-related changes are progressive and will require ever-increasing compensatory measures. The older animal, holding moderate body condition and possibly still in light work, could be expected to have an appetite of approximately 2% of his BM as DM daily (eg, 10 kg of DM for a 500 kg horse). Although appetite remains at this level, 80% (8 kg) of the DM intake should be provided by forage and 2 × 1 kg DM concentrate meals should be adequate.

With time, decreased appetite, and progressive dental loss, the proportion of the diet offered as untreated forage may need to be reduced. Pasture access should still be encouraged, but frequent (3–4 times daily), small meals (1–1.5 kg DM) of dampened compound feeds should be offered; ultimately, it may be essential to change to a processed forage replacer. Total dietary provision should still provide 2% of BM as DM. Horses can be maintained without the inclusion of long fiber, and some compound diets containing ground/pelleted, highly digestible forages are suitable for adaptation as complete diets. Pelleted diets should be thoroughly soaked before feeding and offered as frequent, freshly soaked meals to preserve palatability. Providing a daily mineral and vitamin supplement is a sensible and inexpensive precaution. Continuous access to fresh water is essential.

THE HORSE WITH PITUITARY PARS INTERMEDIA DYSFUNCTION

The nutritional management of confirmed insulin-resistant PPID cases can be problematic. Given the predisposition and potential severity of laminitis in PPID cases, the maintenance of body weight should be accomplished without recourse to cereals or compound feeds and forages high (>10% DM) in NSC.[6] Plasma concentrations of vitamin C (ascorbate) are reduced in these animals, and dietary supplementation is essential. Despite the presence of visible, abnormal fat deposits in many of these animals, increased plasma cortisol concentrations favor catabolic pathways, including muscle atrophy, and the paradoxic deposition of inappropriate fat appears to form an irretrievable loss of useful dietary energy. Although these animals may superficially seem obese in certain body regions, clinical cases are generally in energy deficit.

SUMMARY

Leisure animals now comprise the majority of working horses in industrialized nations; a shift that has decreased workloads yet improved veterinary care and lifetime health. Although many horses now progress well into their 20s without any requirement for dietary modification, age-related changes are insidious, and older animals benefit from regular veterinary monitoring to identify, address, and ameliorate the inevitable onset of age-related disease. Basal metabolic rate decreases with age; older animals expend less energy on controlled exercise, and there can be an increased propensity toward the development of obesity, which needs to be recognized and managed. Conversely, weight loss in elderly animals may be assumed inevitable, yet many of these cases can be managed effectively by appropriate treatment of concurrent disease or correction of management practices. The early recognition of PPID and the onset of senescent changes allow the timely introduction of nutritional interventions.

REFERENCES

1. Wyse CA, McNie KA, Tannahil VJ, et al. Prevalence of obesity in riding horses in Scotland. Vet Rec 2008;162:590–1.

2. Ireland JL, Clegg PD, McGowan CM, et al. A cross-sectional study of geriatric horses in the United Kingdom. Part 1: demographics and management practices. Equine Vet J 2011;43:30–6.

3. McKeever KH, Malinowski K. Exercise capacity in young and geriatric female horses. Am J Vet Res 1997;58:1468–72.

4. Jarvis NG. Nutrition of the aged horse. Vet Clin Equine 2009;25:155–66.

5. Phillips F. Nutrition for healthy ageing. Nutrition Bulletin 2003;28:253–63.

6. McFarlane D. Pathophysiology and clinical features of pituitary pars intermedia dysfunction. Equine Vet Educ 2014;26:592–8.

7. Morrison PK, Bing C, Harris PA, et al. Preliminary investigation into a potential role for myostatin and its receptor (ActRIIB) in lean and obese horses and ponies. PLoS One 2014;9:e112621.

8. Lehnhard RA, McKeever KH, Kearns CF, et al. Myosin heavy chain profiles and body composition are different in old versus young Standardbred mares. Vet J 2004;167:59–66.

9. Kane RA, Fisher M, Parrett D, et al. Estimating fatness in horses. Proceedings of 10th Equine Nutrition and Physiology Society. Fort Collins (CO): 1987. p. 127–31.

10. Argo CM, Dugdale AHA, Morrison PK, et al. Evaluating body composition in living horses: where are we up to?. In: Maltin C, Craigie C, Bünger L, editors. Farm animal imaging III. Copenhagen (Denmark): European Cooperation in Science and Technology; 2014. p. 14–9.

11. McFarlane D. Pituitary pars intermedia dysfunction. Vet Clin Equine 2011;27: 93–113.

12. Brosnahan MM, Paradis MR. Assessment of clinical characteristics, management practices, and activities of geriatric horses. J Am Vet Med Assoc 2003;223: 99–103.

13. Ireland JL, Clegg PD, McGowan CM, et al. A cross-sectional study of geriatric horses in the United Kingdom. Part 2: health care and disease. Equine Vet J 2011;43:37–44.

14. McKeever KH, Eaton TL, Geiser S, et al. Thermoregulation in old and young horses during exercise [abstract]. Med Sci Sports Exerc 2000;32(Suppl):S156.

15. Ralston SL, Harris PA. Nutritional considerations for aged horses. In: Geor RJ, Harris PA, Coenen M, editors. Equine applied and clinical nutrition: health welfare and performance. London: Saunders Elsevier; 2013. p. 289–303.

16. National Academy of Sciences. Dietary references intakes (DRIs) for energy, carbohydrate, fiber, fat, fatty acids, cholesterol, protein, and amino acids. Food and Nutrition Board; Institute of Medicine; Washington, DC: National Academies; 2004.

17. Ireland JL, Clegg PD, McGowan CM, et al. Comparison of owner-reported health problems with veterinary assessment of geriatric horses in the United Kingdom. Equine Vet J 2012;44:94–100.

18. Ireland JL, McGowan CM, Clegg PD, et al. A survey of health care and disease in geriatric horses aged 30 years or older. Vet J 2012;192:57–64.

19. Ralston SL. Digestive alterations in aged horses. Equine Vet Sci 1989;9:203–5.

20. du Toit N, Rucker BA. The gold standard of dental care: the geriatric horse. Vet Clin Equine 2013;29:521–7.

21. Dixon PM, Dacre I. A review of equine dental disorders. Vet J 2005;169:165–87.

22. Appleby MC. Social rank and food access in red deer stags. Behaviour 1980;74: 294–309.

23. Ingólfsdóttir HB, Sigurjónsdóttir H. The benefits of high rank in the wintertime—a study of the Icelandic horse. Appl Anim Behav Sci 2008;114:485–91.

24. Keiper R. Social interactions of the Przewalski horse (Equus prze-walskii Poliakov, 1881) herd at the Munich Zoo. Appl Anim Behav Sci 1988;21:89–97.
25. Rutberg AT, Greenberg SA. Dominance, aggression frequencies and modes of aggressive competition in feral pony mares. Anim Behav 1990;40:322–31.
26. Van Dierendonck MC, De Vries H, Schilder MB. An analysis of dominance, its behavioural parameters and possible determinants in a herd of Icelandic horses in captivity. Neth J Zool 1995;45:362–85.
27. Sigurjónsdóttir H, Van Dierendonck MC, Snorrason S, et al. Social relationships in a group of horses without a mature stallion. Behaviour 2003;140:783–804.
28. Giles SL, Nicole CJ, Harris PA, et al. Dominance rank is associated with body condition in outdoor-living domestic horses (Equus caballus). Appl Anim Behav Sci 2015;166:71–9.
29. Brosnahan MM, Paradis MR. Demographic and clinical characteristics of geriatric horses: 467 cases (1989–1999). J Am Vet Med Assoc 2003;223(1):93–8.
30. Dougal K, de la Fuente G, Harri PA, et al. Characterisation of the Faecal bacterial community in adult and elderly horses fed a high fibre, high oil or high starch diet using 454 pyrosequencing. PLoS One 2014;9:e87424.
31. Biagi E, Nylund L, Candela M, et al. Through ageing, and beyond: gut microbiota and inflammatory status in seniors and centenarians. PLoS One 2010;5:e10667.
32. Rajilic-Stojanovic M, Heilig HGHJ, Molenaar D, et al. Development and application of the human intestinal tract chip, a phylogenetic microarray: analysis of universally conserved phylotypes in the abundant microbiota of young and elderly adults. Environ Microbiol 2009;11:1736–51.
33. Mariat D, Firmesse O, Levenez F, et al. The Firmicutes/Bacteroidetes ration of the human microbiota changes with age. BMC Microbiol 2009;9:123.
34. Dougal K, Harris PA, Edwards A, et al. A comparison of the microbiome and the metabolome of different regions of the equine hindgut. FEMS Microbiol Ecol 2012;82:642–52.
35. Dougal K, de la Fuente G, Harris PA, et al. Identification of a core bacterial community within the large intestine of the horse. PLoS One 2013;8:e77660.
36. Hopkins MJ, MacFarlane GT. Changes in predominant bacterial populations in human faeces with age and with Clostridium difficile infection. J Med Microbiol 2002;52:448–54.
37. Elzinga S, Nielsen BD, Schott HC, et al. Comparison of nutrient digestibility between adult and aged horses. J Equine Vet Sci 2014;34:1164–9.
38. Ralston SL, Squires EL, Nockels CF. Digestion in the aged horse re-visited. Equine Vet Sci 2001;2:310–1.
39. Adams AA, Betancourt A, Barker VD, et al. Comparison of the immunologic response to anthelmintic treatment in old versus middle-aged horses. J Equine Vet Sci 2015;35:873–81.
40. McGowan TW, Pinchbeck GP, McGowan CM. Prevalence, risk factors and clinical signs predictive for equine pituitary pars intermedia dysfunction in aged horses. Equine Vet J 2013;45:74–9.
41. Schott HC 2nd. Pituitary pars intermedia dysfunction: equine Cushing's disease. Vet Clin North Am Equine Pract 2002;18:237–70.
42. Donaldson MT, LaMonte BH, Morresey P, et al. Treatment with pergolide or cyproheptadine of pituitary pars intermedia dysfunction (equine Cushing's disease). J Vet Intern Med 2002;16:742–6.
43. Donaldson MT, Jorgensen AJR, Beech J. Evaluation of suspected pituitary pars intermedia dysfunction in horses with laminitis. J Am Vet Med Assoc 2004;224:1123–7.

44. Couetil L, Paradis MR, Knoll J. Plasma adrenocorticotropin concentration in healthy horses and in horses with clinical signs of hyperadrenocorticism. J Vet Intern Med 1996;10:1–6.

45. Beech J. Tumors of the pituitary gland (pars intermedia). In: Robinson NE, editor. Current therapy in equine medicine. 3rd edition. Missouri: W.B. Saunders; 1987. p. 182–5.

46. van der Kolk JH. Diseases of the pituitary gland including hyperadrenocorticism. In: Watson TD, editor. Metabolic and endocrine problems of the horse. New York: WB Saunders Co; 1998. p. 41–59.

47. Hillyer MH, Taylor FG, Mair TS, et al. Diagnosis of hyperadrenocorticism in the horse. Equine Vet Educ 1992;4:131–4.

48. Rossi ABR, Vergnanini AL. Cellulite: a review. J Eur Acad Dermatol Venereol 2000;14:251–62.

49. Dugdale AHA, Curtis GC, Harris PA, et al. Assessment of body fat in the pony: I. Relationships between the anatomical distribution of adipose tissue, body composition and body condition. Equine Vet J 2011;43:552–61.

50. Dugdale AHA, Grove-White DH, Curtis GC, et al. Body condition scoring as a predictor of body fat in horses and ponies. Vet J 2012;194:173–8.

51. Argo CM, Dugdale AHA, McGowan CM. Management of equine metabolic syndrome and obesity: considerations for the use of restricted, soaked grass hay diets to promote weight loss. Vet J 2015;206:170–7.

52. McGowan CM, Dugdale AH, Pinchbeck GL, et al. Dietary restriction in combination with a nutraceutical supplement for the management of equine metabolic syndrome in horses. Vet J 2013;196:153–9.

53. Argo CM, Curtis GC, Grove-White D, et al. Weight loss resistance; a further consideration for the nutritional management of obese Equidae. Vet J 2012; 194:179–88.

54. Longland AC, Barfoot C, Harris PA. The effect of wearing a grazing muzzle vs not wearing a grazing muzzle on pasture dry matter intake by ponies. J Equine Vet Sci 2011;31:282–3.

55. Dugdale AHA, Curtis GC, Cripps P, et al. Effect of dietary restriction on body condition, composition and welfare of overweight and obese pony mares. Equine Vet J 2010;42(7):600–10.

56. Frank N, Geor RJ, Bailey SR, et al. Equine metabolic syndrome. J Vet Intern Med 2010;24:467–75.

57. Longland AC, Barfoot C, Harris PA. The loss of water-soluble carbohydrate and soluble protein from nine different hays soaked in water for up to 16 hours. J Equine Vet Sci 2009;29:383–4.

58. Bruynsteen L, Janssens GPJ, Harris PA, et al. Changes in oxidative stress in response to different levels of energy restriction in obese ponies. Br J Nutr 2014;112:1402–11.

59. Ralston SL, Squires EL, Nockels CF. Digestion in the aged horse. Equine Vet Sci 1989;9:203–5.

60. Ralston SL, Breuer LH. Field evaluation of a feed formulated for geriatric horses. J Equine Vet Sci 1996;16:334–8.

61. Siciliano PD. Nutrition and feeding of the geriatric horse. Vet Clin Equine 2002;18: 491–508.

62. Ralston SL. Evidence-based equine nutrition. Vet Clin North Am Equine Pract 2007;23:365–84.

Welfare, Quality of Life, and Euthanasia of Aged Horses

Catherine M. McGowan, BVSc, MACVS, PhD, FHEA, MRCVS[a],*,
Joanne L. Ireland, BVMS, PhD, Cert AVP(EM), MRCVS[b]

KEYWORDS

- Geriatric • Human–horse bond • Old age • Grief • Welfare • Mortality

KEY POINTS

- The human–horse bond, strengthened by years of ownership, is strong in geriatric horses and affects owner decision-making about their horses' welfare, quality of life (QoL), and euthanasia.
- Mortality rates increase with increasing age in horses with the overall incidence of mortality in aged horses between 9 to 11 mortalities per 100 horse years at risk.
- Owners of geriatric horses want to maximize the welfare of their horses but may under-recognize clinical signs of disease or attribute them to senescence rather than disease.
- The gastrointestinal and musculoskeletal systems are the most commonly implicated as resulting in death or euthanasia; however, concurrent chronic disease has a major influence on horse owners' decision for euthanasia.
- QoL assessment could play an important role in informing euthanasia decisions. Veterinarians should be proactive in discussing QoL with owners.

INTRODUCTION

The relationship between humans and horses is unique and powerful, with the development of a bond reinforced by years of interaction between owners and their aged horses.[1] Inevitably, owners of geriatric horses will be faced with deteriorating health of their animals as they advance in years. Although all horse owners want to maximize the welfare of their aged horses, owners of geriatric horses may not recognize clinical signs or appreciate their significance, or might mistakenly attribute them to old age.[2] Nonetheless, owners are often the best placed to determine the quality of life (QoL) of

Disclosure Statement: The authors have nothing to disclose.
[a] Faculty of Health and Life Sciences, Institute of Ageing and Chronic Disease, University of Liverpool, Leahurst Campus, Neston, Wirral, CH64 7TE, UK; [b] Epidemiology and Disease Surveillance, Centre for Preventive Medicine, Animal Health Trust, Lanwades Park, Kentford, Newmarket CB8 7UU, Suffolk, UK
* Corresponding author.
E-mail address: C.M.Mcgowan@liverpool.ac.uk

their own horses and, furthermore, are the ones faced with the decision for euthanasia in a horse with a compromised QoL.[3,4] Such a decision is usually far from easy and can be a huge burden on owners, who often rely on advice from their veterinarian. The aim of this article is to outline the role of aged horses, define welfare and QoL of aged horses, and explore causes and experiences of mortality in aged horses.

THE ROLE OF AGED HORSES AND THE HUMAN–HORSE BOND

The role of horses in Western society has changed dramatically during the past century with the decline of the working horse and concurrent proliferation of the performance horse.[5] Such performance activities include anything from recreational riding to racing disciplines. In Western countries, the predominant horse use is for recreation rather than commercial reasons. For example, in the United Kingdom, a recent survey of more than 15,000 horse owners found more than a third of horses were used for leisure and hacking, around a third used mainly for equestrianism (eventing, dressage, show jumping and showing), and a further 20% used for a variety of purposes from racing or breeding to hippotherapy.[6]

However, in the past few decades, even the role of horses as recreational performance animals has been challenged. In the United Kingdom, 12% of horses were not kept for performance and were unridden and/or companions.[6] This supports survey-based research of almost 50,000 households across the United States where 38.4% of horse owners considered their horses to be family members, more than half (56.5%) considered their horses to be a pet or companion, with only 5.1% considering them to be property.[7] In a Dutch survey of horse enthusiasts, 47% respondents indicated that horses were like a partner or child to them.[8] Although these reports are not age-specific, demographic research has shown aged horses typically have similar roles. In survey research of horses 15 or more years of age, approximately 60% of the horses were used for leisure or hacking, whereas 30% to 40% of the horses were retired or kept as a companion.[9,10]

This altered, noncommercial role of horses in Western societies has been reflected in the management of aged horses, in which owners of aged horses that are pets or companions, or even those used for recreation and leisure, have different influences and reasons for management decisions compared with those who keep their animals for commercial reasons. Surveys have shown that horses are being kept into their old age and into retirement; approximately 25% of the horse population is 15 years or older.[10] Although some aspects of health care have been shown to be reduced following retirement, owners are interested in the health and welfare of their aged horses, and the ability to maintain the horses' QoL.[11] Owners of aged horses asked to record their perceptions of health issues they considered important in horses 15 or years or older volunteered welfare, management, and preventive care as important issues, as well as medical or health-related conditions. The most commonly reported were maintaining the horse's condition, arthritis or lameness, teeth or dental care, psychological health (horse "feels" cared for), exercise for health (including not excessive exercise), and protection from the environment (rugging, warmth, shelter).[11] The concern horse owners have for the health and welfare of their aged horses is also reflected in veterinary care, with geriatric horse admissions increasing steadily almost 6-fold from 2.2% of the total equine patient admissions to 12.5% over a 10-year period.[12]

The basis of the role change of horses is likely due to a combination of the relative affluence of many horse owners living in Western countries, as well as the unique and powerful relationship between humans and horses. Most aged horses have been in the owner's possession for more than 10 years,[9,10] with years of interaction between owners and their aged horses reinforcing the bond between them.[1] The relationship between humans and horses is unique compared with production or companion animals. The shared experience of exercise, recreation, competitive sport, or performance forms the basis of a strong relationship of trust, and respect, again strengthened over many years.[1,13,14] For many people, the entire lifestyle of owning a horse is a key factor and an important part of their life. Other factors may include the ability to control such a powerful animal or the feeling of superiority or status when riding.[13] Ultimately the human–horse bond affects owner decision making about their horses' welfare, QoL and euthanasia. This must be considered and acknowledged by veterinarians in making decisions involving treatment or euthanasia of aged horses.

OWNER RESPONSIBILITIES AND AWARENESS OF EQUINE WELFARE

Owners, keepers, and industry professionals have a moral and legal responsibility to care for their horses and to ensure their physical and mental wellbeing.[14] It is the owner's or keeper's responsibility to be able to recognize ill health and seek veterinary assistance as required, and to recognize when QoL deteriorates, seek veterinary advice if necessary and arrange euthanasia when appropriate.[15] Despite clear intent to maximize the welfare of their aged horses, owners of geriatric horses may under-recognize clinical signs of disease, possibly mistakenly regarding these changes as senescence rather than attributing them to disease.[2,11,16–18] This could result in owners electing not to seek appropriate veterinary attention and possibly compromising the welfare of their aging horse.

As well as appropriate recognition, seeking advice from appropriate sources is important for equine welfare. Among United Kingdom horse owners, veterinarians and farriers were reported to be the most frequent source of equine health information.[19] In another survey undertaken in the Netherlands, 75% of horse owners sought equine health and management advice from their veterinarian, with 55% seeking information regarding equine welfare; however, welfare was the second most frequent topic for which owners reported difficulty in obtaining information.[8] Owner awareness of factors that can negatively impact equine welfare does not necessarily translate to their utilization of appropriate management practices.[8] In a small survey of Australian Pony Club members, 84% of owners considered their veterinarian to be an important factor in their horse's health, yet 19% reported learning about equine health through trial and error, and only 9% stated that they would always consult their veterinarian for advice on horse health.[20] Somewhat alarmingly, increased owner reliance on the Internet as an advice source was identified as a major factor in declining companion animal veterinary visits.[21] If their pet was sick or injured, 39% of companion animal owners reported that they would seek medical information online in the first instance, with 15% of owners indicating that they relied less on their veterinarian because of readily available information on the Internet.[21] Should a similar trend occur among horse owners, reduced veterinary involvement in the care of geriatric horses could have considerable impact on their health and welfare.

QUALITY OF LIFE

Although QoL is a term used extensively in both human and veterinary health care, a single consistent definition is lacking.[22] QoL is often considered synonymously with welfare when referring to animals.[23–25] However, the concept of QoL seems to have a different emphasis to welfare, encompassing both pleasant and unpleasant feelings,[26] and incorporating physical health, psychological state, and general enjoyment of life.[24,27,28]

Assessing Quality of Life

QoL assessment is well established in human geriatric medicine,[29] with specific assessment tools validated for monitoring the effect of pain, chronic diseases, and age-related changes on QoL.[30–32] QoL assessments are also used to evaluate the success of medical treatment or other interventions,[33] and have been reported as useful prognostic indicators in geriatric patients with neoplastic conditions.[34,35]

Use of a questionnaire with well-established reliability and validity is considered to be the gold standard in QoL assessment[36]; however, there is limited information regarding equine QoL assessment and no validated instrument is currently available in equine medicine. As in human patients, geriatric horses are more likely to suffer from chronic disease,[11,16,17,37,38] and with increasing age they are less likely to receive routine veterinary attention and preventive health care measures.[11,17] Therefore, it is likely that aged horses have different welfare requirements and dissimilar factors influencing their QoL compared with younger animals.

QoL assessment tools, focused on health-related QoL for specific conditions or diseases, have been developed for use in small animal medicine.[39–42] Less common are questionnaires not specific for disease but for the general assessment of physical and mental well-being, with some developed for use in dogs[23,43,44], and cats.[45] Other forms of welfare assessment tools have been developed for production livestock species.[46,47] However, the welfare requirements of horses clearly differ from those of small animals and livestock; therefore, direct extrapolation of previously published tools for these species is not possible for equine QoL assessment.

Health status is frequently equated with QoL, being a primary focus of veterinary assessments[25,48] and the most widely accepted contributing factor.[49] In human geriatric medicine, ill health has been used as a proxy measure of QoL,[50] and there is greater agreement between proxies and patients for the assessment of more observable health states.[51] Although health necessarily continues to be an important determinant of QoL, in isolation it is not considered to be a sufficient proxy among elderly human patients.[31] Patients with significant health problems do not necessarily have QoL ratings proportionate with their health,[52] and suffering from chronic disease does not necessarily lead to poor QoL in geriatric humans, with other factors contributing to patients' rating of their QoL.[53]

Existing tools for evaluation of equine welfare focus on environmental assessment or indicators of health status, including body condition score (BCS), hydration status, pain or lameness scales, and cardiorespiratory parameters, as reviewed by Hockenhull and Whay.[54] Although these parameters may provide some measure of health-related QoL, assessment of single or combined health indicators alone is unlikely to be sufficient in evaluating equine geriatric QoL. For example, both weight loss and obesity are prevalent in geriatric horses,[11,17,55] and, although they may affect morbidity and mortality risk,[56] the effect of BCS on equine QoL has not been evaluated.

There has been a shift towards obtaining individualized QoL assessments in human medicine, asking patients to identify those areas of life or life activities they consider most important in terms of their own QoL. This approach would be readily transferable to veterinary medicine, and an owner-perceived QoL assessment method has been reported for use in dogs.[57] In clinical settings, a rapid evaluation comprising a short series of single-item questions can be used to provide valid QoL assessment, allowing identification of individuals with poor QoL requiring further evaluation.[36] Together with a thorough veterinary examination, asking owners to identify QoL domains that they consider to be important for their geriatric horse could be a useful way to inform a tailored, single-item question format, assessment for rating and monitoring QoL in that individual.

The Role of the Owner in Quality of Life Assessment

In human medicine, patient self-assessment questionnaires are favored because they gather information about an individual's perspective or subjective feelings directly from that individual. This is clearly not possible in veterinary medicine because assessment of QoL can only be performed by a human observer reporting on behalf of the animal.[45,58] Most frequently, veterinarians will evaluate equine welfare at individual animal level,[54] and QoL assessment performed by a veterinarian is often the most practical proxy measure. Clinician-based observation can be considerably less time consuming than patient interviews or questionnaire completion in human medicine.[59] However, physician QoL ratings have been reported to show poor agreement with patient ratings,[53,60] with physicians underestimating QoL in geriatric humans.[53] Proxies may overestimate health limitations, particularly for less observable health constructs such as emotions and mental status.[51] It is probable that this effect will be even more significant in equine medicine, in which a single clinical examination is unlikely to result in a complete, reliable assessment of the horse's QoL in its normal environment, performing a full range of activities.

Although veterinarians may be more effective assessors of equine health, owners have more experience of the individual horse[49] and may be in a better position to assess mental well-being and experience. Duration of ownership for geriatric horses tends to be prolonged,[9,10,16,37] and most owners are responsible for the daily care of their geriatric horse.[10] Compared with veterinarians, owners have considerably greater knowledge of their animal's history and normal daily activities. Therefore, owners can be useful proxies for QoL assessments as they are familiar with their animal's character, behavior, and daily routine,[61] and have an increased awareness of the importance of external factors from the individual animal's perspective.[62] Research involving geriatric horses has shown that owners are well placed to assess the QoL of their own horses.[3]

Rating of QoL relies on the individual's perception and interpretation, with the potential for several forms of introduced personal bias.[63] There are, therefore, some concerns that using owners as proxies for animal QoL assessment may be unreliable due to the subjective nature of such assessments.[58] Owner's perceptions of QoL and factors influencing it are likely to be affected by some degree of anthropomorphism or anthropocentrism. To assess their animal's QoL, owners must be able to recognize factors affecting QoL and interpret the effect these factors have on their animal's well-being, without superimposing their own feelings.[64]

Therefore, it seems that a comprehensive assessment of equine geriatric QoL should involve both the owner or caregiver and the veterinarian. This approach is also likely to yield further benefits. Integrating QoL assessments during routine veterinary examinations could help engage clients in conversations that would increase their understanding of the importance of regular veterinary care.[58] It would also provide an opportunity to assess the owner's perceptions of health problems and treatment options, and to identify concerns that have not been apparent to the owner.[62] Of particular importance in equine geriatric medicine, regular QoL discussions could serve to increase owner awareness of factors affecting their aged horse's QoL and to encourage owners to consider geriatric health concerns, provision of analgesia if appropriate, and routine preventive health care measures such as parasite control and weight management.[62]

Factors Affecting Quality of Life in Geriatric Horses

Almost all owners consider their geriatric horses to have good or excellent QoL; however, increasing horse age is associated with reduced owner QoL rating.[3] Welfare issues were ranked as the fourth most important health issue affecting geriatric horses in a large survey of Australian owners[11] and among horse owners in the Netherlands, 99.6% stated that good health is an indicator of good welfare.[8] It is, therefore, unsurprising that existing health problems had a negative association with owner-assessed QoL, and increasing horse age corresponded negatively with several health-related QoL factors in geriatric horses.[3] Improved health or successful management or treatment of a chronic disease was the most frequently reported (18%) single important change that owners considered would improve the QoL of their geriatric horse.[3] QoL is also a highly important consideration in owner decision-making regarding treatment options or euthanasia.[3]

Although health status plays a major role in owner assessment of equine geriatric QoL, management factors, such as nutrition, comfort, and company of other horses, were stated as important factors influencing QoL by a greater proportion of owners than health-related factors such as preventive health care and effective analgesia.[3] Nutritional or dietary requirements were the most numerous factors considered by owners to be influential in equine geriatric QoL,[3] and comfort (eg, stabling, shelter, warmth, rugs) is also considered to be a highly important factor.[3,11] Companionship is an important aspect of QoL for prey animals that naturally live in small social groups, such as the horse, and this seems to be well recognized by owners of geriatric horses.[3,11] Owners also indicated that factors relating to exercise (ie, attention to concurrent health problems; regular exercise routine; frequency, intensity, and variety of exercise; and sympathetic riding) are important in maintaining their geriatric horse's QoL.[3,11] Exercise is considered to be a pleasurable experience that has a positive effect on QoL in dogs,[23,65] and it is likely that owners of geriatric horses have an equivalent perception. However, owners seem to under-recognize lameness in aged horses,[11,18] and considerable proportion of geriatric horses exhibiting lameness on veterinary examination are still involved in athletic activities.[55]

Activities of daily living (ADL) are key components in QoL assessment in human geriatric patients,[66] and lower scores for several owner-assessed ADL measures were associated with an increased risk of mortality in geriatric horses.[56] Although increasing age may certainly have a negative effect on the ability to perform daily activities, it is possible that owners of geriatric horses will accept some degree of limitation as a normal aging effect,[11,17] whereas in a younger animal this might be interpreted as an indication of pain or disease.

CAUSES OF MORTALITY AND EUTHANASIA IN GERIATRIC HORSES

Unsurprisingly, mortality rates increase with increasing age in geriatric horses.[56,67,68] The overall incidence of mortality in aged horses has been reported as between 9 to 11 mortalities per 100 horse years at risk, with the rate of 4 to 6 per 100 horse years at risk for horses aged 15 to 20 years increasing to 35 to 42 per 100 horse years at risk for animals older than 30 years.[56,68]

Causes of mortality and reasons for euthanasia in aged horses varying depending on whether owner reported or the result of postmortem examination. Veterinary-reported causes of mortality and reasons for euthanasia in aged horses are largely similar between studies, with some variation depending on the study population. At postmortem examination of horses 15 years or older in the breeding region of Kentucky, the most common body system implicated as resulting in death was the gastrointestinal, followed by the musculoskeletal and reproductive systems.[69] When horses older than 20 years were separated, the most common individual diagnoses were neoplasia and pituitary pars intermedia dysfunction (PPID).[69] Similarly in horses 15 years or older undergoing postmortem examination from a referral hospital, death was most commonly attributed to the gastrointestinal system, followed by PPID and the locomotor system, with neoplastic disease as a cause of death increasing from 16% in horses 15 to 20 years, to 22% in horses older than 20 years.[70]

Within the equine geriatric population, the most common reasons for euthanasia were similar to those from hospital postmortem reports but with lameness most commonly reported, followed by colic; in agreement with previous studies of the general equine population.[71–73] Musculoskeletal disorders are an important cause of death in horses of all ages[67,72]; however, geriatric horses are more likely to have a nontraumatic cause of fatal locomotor disease,[74] with a low prevalence of fatal limb fractures reported in animals aged 15 years or older.[56] Musculoskeletal disease in owner-reported surveys may not be a direct cause of death of aged horses but may be a reason for euthanasia. Similarly, owners also listed nonspecific chronic disease (chronic illness[56] or weight loss[68]) as a reason for euthanasia, either concurrently or primarily. Weight loss was the second most common reason for euthanasia of aged horses in Australia[68] and, compared with animals considered by their owner to be in good body condition, underweight geriatric horses were at increased risk of mortality.[56]

Owners seem to take into consideration concurrent disease, evidence of senescence, and debilitation ("old age"), as well as specific diagnoses. In an owner survey, 26.8% of all equine euthanasia was reported to be performed due to a combination of old age and concurrent disease, with a further 8.4% due to "old-age difficulties" and 4.2% were a result of a combination of old age and accidental injury.[75] Similarly, the US Department of Agriculture's National Animal Health Monitoring System's Equine report found that, "old age" was listed as the most common identified cause of death or euthanasia in horses older than 6 months of age (29% of deaths), and more than two-thirds of deaths in horses aged 20 years or older.[76] Old age was also reported as the most common reason for horses becoming nonambulatory (unable to stand or rise on its own without assistance, or able to stand but not able to walk), with 10.4% of horses aged 30 years or older reported to become nonambulatory within the previous year.[67] In addition to being an important cause of mortality, inability to ambulate is also a considerable welfare concern.

Though old age cannot be considered a specific cause of death or euthanasia, it may represent an owner's justification for euthanasia of an aged horse. It suggests that increasing horse age or senescence may influence owners' decisions regarding treatment options for their older horses. The cost of keeping a retired geriatric horse or the expense of treatment of concurrent disease may make an owner more likely to opt for euthanasia than to embark on expensive or prolonged treatment of an additional health problem. In cases in which geriatric horses had concurrent diseases, 43% of owners stated that this existing health problem influenced their decision-making regarding euthanasia, whereas only 2% of owners reported that financial considerations influenced their decision to euthanize.[56] Similarly, economic factors were infrequently stated as a reason for euthanasia of aged horses in Australia.[68]

EXPERIENCES OF MORTALITY AND EUTHANASIA IN GERIATRIC HORSES

Almost all owners of geriatric horses are inevitably going to be faced with a decision of euthanasia in their horse at some point and it is important to consider the implications of the conflicting pressures faced by owners of aged horses in making this decision. Most aged horses are euthanized,[56,68] with veterinarians performing euthanasia in most cases.[56] Owners consider euthanasia of their horse to be a difficult decision[4] and consider the advice of their veterinarian to be important in making the decision.[4,56,77–79] Owners asked to rank factors that influenced their decision to euthanize their horse ranked veterinary advice and conditions that had a hopeless prognosis or caused incurable, recurrent, or acute severe pain as most important.[3,4] However, the owner's relationship with the horse and anticipated quality of the horse's life were equally ranked, emphasizing the importance of the human–horse bond and the concern owners of aged horses have towards the welfare of their horses.[4]

As well as being a difficult decision to make, most horse owners report that the loss of their horse is a distressing experience.[4,78] Although the act of euthanasia itself can be a particularly stressful or shocking event for an owner, especially in an emergency situation,[13] research has found that the degree of distress to owners caused by the loss of an aged horse was greater on a visual analog scale than the degree of distress caused by the actual procedure of euthanasia.[4] However, in cases in which the actual procedure was perceived as less acceptable, there was a correlation with a more distressing experience.[4] Other research has shown that owners commonly feel grief for many months to years after euthanasia of their horse, comparable to that experienced by companion animal owners following the loss of their pet.[78,80] Owners who spent a longer period of time per day with their horse or who had experienced an unpleasant euthanasia of their horse had a significantly longer grieving period.[78]

The personality of the horse owner can also affect the degree of distress or grief felt following euthanasia of their horse. Horse owners who found the decision to euthanize their aged horse particularly hard scored higher in the domain of neuroticism, using a five-factor personality model, than those who found the decision a major but less difficult decision.[4] This might indicate those owners who found the decision more difficult had a greater sense of apprehension, a tendency to experience states of frustration and bitterness, and would be susceptible to experiencing guilt, sadness, and loneliness.[4] Although all owners are likely to benefit from grief counseling,[77] identifying owners susceptible to such negative feelings may be particularly important. A good explanation of the procedure, active support by the veterinarian after the euthanasia, and a good relationship between the veterinarian and the owner have all been associated with better owner experiences of euthanasia.[78]

There are many factors that may influence an owner faced with the decision to euthanize their horse, including their own personality and experiences of euthanasia in the past and the strength of relationship with their horse.[4] Despite an owner's best intentions, the welfare of aged horses can be as compromised by delaying euthanasia due to fears about doing the best thing for the animal or the perceived distress it will cause them or their family, as those owners who compromise welfare by simply neglecting their aged horse.[5] There is evidence that improvement in communication by the veterinarian before, during, and after the actual event of euthanasia can help support owners, especially those who are finding the decision very difficult.[4,77,78] QoL assessment could play an important role in informing euthanasia decisions, and if veterinarians are proactive in discussing QoL with owners, there is an opportunity to ensure that the owner is better prepared for making the decision to euthanize when the time comes.[79]

SUMMARY

Owners of geriatric horses frequently have a very strong bond with their aged animal, which can influence their perceptions of welfare and QoL and their decisions involving treatment options or euthanasia. Evaluating health status alone is insufficient for the comprehensive assessment of QoL, and owners are well placed to assess the QoL of their own geriatric horses, considering several factors not related to health are important to their animal's QoL. Mortality rates increase with increasing age in geriatric horses and most aged horses are euthanized by veterinarians. Musculoskeletal disorders, colic, and chronic disease are the most common reasons for euthanasia; however, in addition to specific diagnoses, horse age, senescence, debilitation, and concurrent disease also influence owner decision-making. Horse owners find reaching the decision to euthanize their horse difficult, and the loss of their aged horse is a distressing experience. The degree of distress or grief felt following euthanasia of their horse is influenced by the strength of the human–horse bond and by the owner's personality. Increased veterinary involvement in QoL assessment and greater client communication regarding euthanasia could improve equine geriatric welfare and help to support owners facing this difficult decision.

REFERENCES

1. Estep DQ. Interactions with horses and the human-animal bond. In: Bertone JJ, editor. Equine geriatric medicine and surgery. St Louis (MO): WB Saunders; 2006. p. 5–10.
2. Ireland JL, McGowan CM, Clegg PD, et al. A survey of health care and disease in geriatric horses aged 30 years or older. Vet J 2012;192(1):57–64.
3. Ireland JL, Clegg PD, McGowan CM, et al. Owners' perceptions of quality of life in geriatric horses: a cross-sectional study. Anim Welf 2011;20:483–95.
4. McGowan TW, Phillips CJ, Hodgson DR, et al. Euthanasia in aged horses: relationship between the owner's personality and their opinions on, and experience of, euthanasia of horses. Anthrozoös 2012;25(3):261–75.
5. McGowan C. Welfare of aged horses. Animals (Basel) 2011;1(4):366–76.
6. Slater J. National Equine Health Survey (NEHS) 2015, Blue Cross, 12th August 2015. www.bluecross.org.uk/. Accessed December 8, 2015.
7. Pet ownership & demographics sourcebook. Schaumburg (IL): American Veterinary Medical Association; 2007. p. 39–44, 210-124.
8. Visser EK, Van Wijk-Jansen EEC. Diversity in horse enthusiasts with respect to horse welfare: an explorative study. J Vet Behav 2012;7:295–304.
9. McGowan TW, Pinchbeck GL, Phillips C, et al. A survey of aged horses in Queensland, Australia. Part 1: management and preventive health care. Aust Vet J 2010;88:420–7.
10. Ireland JL, Clegg PD, McGowan CM, et al. A cross-sectional study of geriatric horses in the United Kingdom. Part 1: Demographics and management practices. Equine Vet J 2011;43:30–6.
11. McGowan TW, Pinchbeck GL, Phillips C, et al. A survey of aged horses in Queensland, Australia. Part 2: clinical signs and owner perceptions of health and welfare. Aust Vet J 2010;88:465–71.
12. Traub-Dargatz JL, Long RE, Bertone JJ. What is an "old horse" and its recent impact?. In: Bertone JJ, editor. Equine geriatric medicine and surgery. St Louis (MO): WB Saunders; 2006. p. 1–4.
13. Brackenridge SS. The human/horse bond and client bereavement in equine practice, part 1. Equine Pract 1996;18:19–22.

14. Hemsworth LM, Jongman E, Coleman GL. Recreational horse welfare: The relationships between recreational horse owner attributes and recreational horse welfare. Appl Anim Behav Sci 2015;165:1–16.
15. Anon. Equine industry welfare guidelines compendium for horses, ponies and donkey. 2nd edition. Banbury (United Kingdom): National Equine Welfare Council; 2005.
16. Brosnahan MM, Paradis MR. Assessment of clinical characteristics, management practices, and activities of geriatric horses. J Am Vet Med Assoc 2003;223: 99–103.
17. Ireland JL, Clegg PD, McGowan CM, et al. A cross-sectional study of geriatric horses in the United Kingdom. Part 2: Health care and disease. Equine Vet J 2011;43:37–44.
18. Ireland JL, Clegg PD, McGowan CM, et al. Comparison of owner-reported health problems with veterinary assessment of geriatric horses in the United Kingdom. Equine Vet J 2012;44:94–100.
19. Hockenhull J, Creighton E. A brief note on the information-seeking behaviour of UK leisure horse owners. J Vet Behav 2013;8:106–10.
20. Buckley P, Dunn T, More SJ. Owners' perceptions of the health and performance of Pony Club horses in Australia. Prev Vet Med 2004;63:121–33.
21. Volk JO, Felsted KE, Thomas JG, et al. Executive summary of the Bayer veterinary care usage study. J Am Vet Med Assoc 2011;238:1275–82.
22. Rapley MA. Life of quality – just what does QOL mean?. In: Quality of life research. London: SAGE Publications Ltd; 2003. p. 26–63.
23. Wojciechowska JI, Hewson CJ, Stryhn H, et al. Development of a discriminative questionnaire to assess nonphysical aspects of quality of life of dogs. Am J Vet Res 2005;66:1453–60.
24. Broom DM. Quality of life means welfare: how is it related to other concepts and assessed? Anim Welf 2007;16(S):45–53.
25. Taylor KD, Mills DS. Is quality of life a useful concept for companion animals? Anim Welf 2007;16(S):55–65.
26. McMillan FD. Maximizing quality of life in ill animals. J Am Anim Hosp Assoc 2003;39:227–35.
27. Sandøe P. Animal and human welfare: are they the same kind of thing? Acta Agricult Scand 1996;27(S):11–5.
28. Saxena S, Orley J. Quality of life assessment: the World Health Organization perspective. Eur Psychiatry 1997;12:263S–6S.
29. Haywood KL, Garratt AM, Fitzpatrick R. Quality of life in older people: a structured review of generic self-assessed health instruments. Qual Life Res 2005; 14:1651–68.
30. Schlenk EA, Erlen JA, Dunbar-Jacob J, et al. Health-related quality of life in chronic disorders: a comparison across studies using the MOS SF-36. Qual Life Res 1998;7:57–65.
31. Hyde M, Wiggins RD, Higgs P, et al. A measure of quality of life in early old age: the theory, development and properties of a needs satisfaction model (CASP-19). Aging Ment Health 2003;7:186–94.
32. Osborne RH, Hawthorne G, Lew EA, et al. Validation of the assessment of quality of life (AQoL) instrument and comparison with the SF-36. J Clin Epidemiol 2003; 56:138–47.
33. Skevington SM, Carse MS, Williams AC. Validation of the WHOQOL-100: pain management improves quality of life for chronic pain patients. Clin J Pain 2001; 17:264–75.

34. Maione P, Perrone F, Gallo C, et al. Pretreatment quality of life and functional status assessment significantly predict survival of elderly patients with advanced non-small-cell lung cancer receiving chemotherapy: a prognostic analysis of the multicenter Italian lung cancer in the elderly study. J Clin Oncol 2005;23: 6865–72.

35. Deschler B, Ihorst G, Platzbecker U, et al. Parameters detected by geriatric and quality of life assessment in 195 older patients with myelodysplastic syndromes and acute myeloid leukemia are highly predictive for outcome. Haematologica 2013;98:208–16.

36. Varricchio CG, Estwing Ferrans C. Quality of life assessments in clinical practice. Semin Oncol Nurs 2010;26:12–7.

37. Chandler KJ, Mellor DJ. A pilot study of the prevalence of disease within a geriatric horse population. In: Proceedings of the 40th Congress of the British Equine Veterinary Association. Newmarket (Canada): Equine Vet J Ltd.; 2001. p. 217.

38. Brosnahan MM, Paradis MR. Demographic and clinical characteristics of geriatric horses: 467 cases (1989-1999). J Am Vet Med Assoc 2003;223:93–8.

39. Hartmann K, Kuffer M. Karnofsky's score modified for cats. Eur J Med Res 1998; 3:95–8.

40. Wiseman-Orr ML, Nolan AM, Reid J, et al. Development of a questionnaire to measure the effects of chronic pain on health-related quality of life in dogs. Am J Vet Res 2004;65:1077–84.

41. Freeman LM, Rush JE, Oyama MA, et al. Development and evaluation of a questionnaire for assessment of health-related quality of life in cats with cardiac disease. J Am Vet Med Assoc 2012;240:1188–93.

42. Wessmann A, Volk HA, Parkin T, et al. Evaluation of quality of life in dogs with idiopathic epilepsy. J Vet Intern Med 2014;28:510–4.

43. Schneider TR. Methods for assessing companion animal quality of life. In: Proceedings of the 2005 North American Veterinary Congress. Orlando, Florida, USA, January 8–12, 2005. p. 443–4.

44. Mullan S, Main D. Preliminary evaluation of a quality of life screening programme for pet dogs. J Small Anim Pract 2007;48:314–22.

45. Bijsmans ES, Jepson RE, Syme HM, et al. Psychometric validation of a general health quality of life tool for cats used to compare healthy cats and cats with chronic kidney disease. J Vet Intern Med 2015;30(1):183–91.

46. Anon. FAWC updates the five freedoms. Vet Rec 1992;131:357.

47. Whay HR, Main DCJ, Green LE, et al. Assessment of the welfare of dairy cattle using animal-based measurements: direct observations and investigation of farm records. Vet Rec 2003;153:197–202.

48. Hewson CJ. Can we assess welfare? Can Vet J 2003;44:749–53.

49. McMillan FD. Quality of life in animals. J Am Vet Med Assoc 2000;216:1904–10.

50. Bowling A. Measuring health. A review of quality of life measurement scales. 2nd edition. Buckingham (United Kingdom): Open University Press; 2001.

51. Haywood KL, Garratt AM, Schmidt LJ, et al. Health status and quality of life in older people: a structured review of patient-reported health instruments report from the Patient-reported Health Instruments Group (formerly the Patient-assessed Health Outcomes Programme) to the Department of Health. 2004. Available at: http://phi.uhce.ox.ac.uk/pdf/phig_older_people_report.pdf. Accessed December 8, 2015.

52. Carr AJ, Higginson IJ. Measuring quality of life: are quality of life measures patient centred? BMJ 2001;322:1357–60.

53. Pearlman RA, Uhlmann RF. Quality of life in chronic diseases: perceptions of elderly patients. J Gerontol 1988;43:M25–30.

54. Hockenhull J, Whay HR. A review of approaches to assessing equine welfare. Equine Vet Educ 2014;26:159–66.

55. Ireland JL, Clegg PD, McGowan CM, et al. Disease prevalence in geriatric horses in the United Kingdom: veterinary clinical assessment of 200 cases. Equine Vet J 2012;44:101–6.

56. Ireland JL, Clegg PD, McGowan CM, et al. Factors associated with mortality of geriatric horses in the United Kingdom. Prev Vet Med 2011;101:204–18.

57. Budke CM, Levine JM, Kerwin SC, et al. Evaluation of a questionnaire for obtaining owner-perceived, weighted quality-of-life assessments for dogs with spinal cord injury. J Am Vet Med Assoc 2008;233:925–30.

58. Spofford N, Lefebvre SL, McCune S, et al. Should the veterinary profession invest in developing methods to assess quality of life in healthy dogs and cats? J Am Vet Med Assoc 2013;243:952–6.

59. Aaronson NK. Quality of life assessment in clinical trials: methodologic issues. Control Clin Trials 1989;10:195S–208S.

60. Schag CC, Heinrich RL, Ganz PA. Karnofsky performance status revisited: reliability, validity and guidelines. J Clin Oncol 1984;2:187–93.

61. Wojciechowska JI, Hewson CJ. Quality-of-life assessment in pet dogs. J Am Vet Med Assoc 2005;226:722–8.

62. Yeates J, Main D. Assessment of companion animal quality of life in veterinary practice and research. J Small Anim Pract 2009;50:274–81.

63. Wemelsfelder F. How animals communicate quality of life: the qualitative assessment of behaviour. Anim Welf 2007;16(S):25–31.

64. Bradshaw JC, Casey RA. Anthropomorphism and anthropocentrism as influences in the quality of life of companion animals. Anim Welf 2007;16(S):149–54.

65. Wiseman ML, Nolan AM, Reid J, et al. Preliminary study on owner-reported behaviour changes associated with chronic pain in dogs. Vet Rec 2001;149: 423–4.

66. Urciuoli O, Dello Buono M, Padoani W, et al. Assessment of quality of life in the oldest-olds living in nursing homes and at home. Arch Gerontol Geriatr 1998; 6(S):507–14.

67. Anon. USDA/APHIS Part 1: baseline reference of equine health and management. Fort Collins (CO): National Animal Health Monitoring System; 2005. p. 1–60.

68. McGowan, T.W., Perkins, N.R., Pinchbeck, G.L., et al. Survival rates of horses In Queensland, Australia over a 2 year period. In: Proceedings of the 11th International Symposium on Veterinary Epidemiology and Economics; 2006.

69. Williams N. Disease conditions in geriatric horses. Equine Pract 2000;22:32.

70. Miller MA, Moore GE, Bertin FR, et al. What's new in old horses? Postmortem diagnoses in mature and aged equids. Vet Pathol 2015;53(2):390–8.

71. Stevens KB, Marr CM, Horn JNR, et al. Effect of left-sided valvular regurgitation on mortality and causes of death among a population of middle-aged and older horses. Vet Rec 2009;164:6–10.

72. Baker JR, Ellis CE. A survey of post-mortem findings in 480 horses 1958 to 1980: (1) Causes of death. Equine Vet J 1981;13:43–6.

73. Egenvall A, Penell JC, Bonnett BN, et al. Mortality of Swedish horses with complete life insurance between 1997 and 2000: variations with sex, age, breed and diagnosis. Vet Rec 2006;158:397–406.

74. Leblond A, Villard I, Leblond L, et al. A retrospective evaluation of the causes of death of 448 insured French horses in 1995. Vet Res Commun 2000;24:85–102.

75. Haydon-Williams LP. An investigation into perceptions and attitudes to equine euthanasia [MSc Thesis]. United Kingdom: University of Central Lancashire; 2001.
76. Anon. 1998 USDA/APHIS Part 1: Baseline reference of equine health and management. Fort Collins (CO): National Animal Health Monitoring System; 1998.
77. Butler C, Lagoni L. Euthanasia and grief support in an equine bond-centered practice. In: Bertone JJ, editor. Equine geriatric medicine and surgery. St Louis (MO): WB Saunders; 2006. p. 231–43.
78. Endenburg N, Kirpensteijn J, Sanders N. Equine euthanasia: the veterinarian's role in providing owner support. Anthrozoös 1999;12:138–41.
79. Rollins BE. Euthanasia and quality of life. J Am Vet Med Assoc 2006;228:1014–6.
80. Scantlebury CE. The epidemiology of equine recurrent colic and horse-owners' lay beliefs and practices regarding colic management and prevention [PhD Thesis]. The University of Liverpool; 2012.

Index

Vet Clin Equine 32 (2016) 369–378
http://dx.doi.org/10.1016/S0749-0739(16)30020-7
0749-0739/16/$ – see front matter
vetequine.theclinics.com

Moving?

Make sure your subscription moves with you!

To notify us of your new address, find your **Clinics Account Number** (located on your mailing label above your name), and contact customer service at:

Email: journalscustomerservice-usa@elsevier.com

800-654-2452 (subscribers in the U.S. & Canada)
314-447-8871 (subscribers outside of the U.S. & Canada)

Fax number: 314-447-8029

Elsevier Health Sciences Division
Subscription Customer Service
3251 Riverport Lane
Maryland Heights, MO 63043

*To ensure uninterrupted delivery of your subscription,
please notify us at least 4 weeks in advance of move.

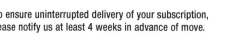

Printed and bound by CPI Group (UK) Ltd, Croydon, CR0 4YY

07/10/2024

01040504-0017